Data Analytics for Pandemics

Pandemics

A COVID-19 Case Study

Intelligent Signal Processing and Data Analysis

Series Editor: Nilanjan Dey

Intelligent signal processing (ISP) methods are progressively swapping the conventional analog signal processing techniques in several domains, such as speech analysis and processing, biomedical signal analysis radar and sonar signal processing, and processing, telecommunications, and geophysical signal processing. The main focus of this book series is to find out the new trends and techniques in the intelligent signal processing and data analysis leading to scientific breakthroughs in applied applications. Artificial fuzzy logic, deep learning, optimization algorithms, and neural networks are the main themes.

Bio-Inspired Algorithms in PID Controller Optimization

Jagatheesan Kallannan, Anand Baskaran, Nilanjan Dey, Amira S. Ashour

A Beginner's Guide to Image Preprocessing Techniques

Jyotismita Chaki, Nilanjan Dey

Digital Image Watermarking: Theoretical and Computational Advances

Surekha Borra, Rohit Thanki, Nilanjan Dey

A Beginner's Guide to Image Shape Feature Extraction Techniques

Jyotismita Chaki, Nilanjan Dey

Coefficient of Variation and Machine Learning Applications

K. Hima Bindu, Raghava Morusupalli, Nilanjan Dey, C. Raghavendra Rao

Data Analytics for Coronavirus Disease (COVID-19) Outbreak

Gitanjali Rahul Shinde, Asmita Balasaheb Kalamkar, Parikshit Narendra Mahalle, Nilanjan Dey

A Beginner's Guide to Multi-Level Image Thresholding

Venkatesan Rajinikanth, Nadaradjane Sri Madhava Raja, Nilanjan Dey

Hybrid Image Processing Methods for Medical Image Examination

Venkatesan Rajinikanth, E. Priya, Hong Lin, Fuhua (Oscar) Lin

For more information about this series, please visit: https://www.routledge.com/Intelligent-Signal-Processing-and-Data-Analysis/book-series/INSPDA

Data Analytics for Pandemics

A COVID-19 Case Study

Gitanjali Rahul Shinde
Asmita Balasaheb Kalamkar
Parikshit N. Mahalle
Nilanjan Dey

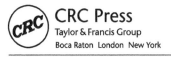

CRC Press
Taylor & Francis Group
Boca Raton London New York

CRC Press is an imprint of the
Taylor & Francis Group, an **informa** business

First edition published 2021
by CRC Press
6000 Broken Sound Parkway NW, Suite 300, Boca Raton, FL 33487-2742

and by CRC Press
2 Park Square, Milton Park, Abingdon, Oxon, OX14 4RN

ISBN: 9780367558468 (hbk)
ISBN: 9781003095415 (ebk)

Typeset in Times
by Deanta Global Publishing Services, Chennai, India

CONTENTS

PREFACE

"**Reshape yourself through the power of your will; never let yourself be degraded by self-will. The will is the only friend of the Self, and the will is the only enemy of the Self.**"

Bhagwad Gita

This book presents an overview of the recent pandemic of COVID-19 and the role of data analytics in such a pandemic for better predictions and forecasting. COVID-19 has a zoonotic origin, i.e. virus being transmitted from animals to human. Symptoms of COVID-19 range from a person showing no signs (asymptomatic) to a person having a severe case of pneumonia. Wuhan, China was the first city to experience the outbreak of COVID-19. The key to understanding the pandemic starts with an understanding of the disease itself, and the progression of the natural course of the disease. The main objective of this book is to present how machine learning techniques can be useful for accurate data analytics, essentially in the context of the recent COVID-19 pandemic. This book presents the different categories of the disease and various ways of disease transmissions. The study of a past pandemic can help us understand the rate of transmission, loss of human life, and nature of the disease. In this view, various past pandemics and stages of the pandemics are discussed in this book.

Accurate prediction of spread and infection rate can help to minimize this outbreak by taking precautionary measures. However, for forecasting, data is required and there are various challenges of data processing. This book presents COVID-19 data sources and their challenges. Techniques for extracting knowledge from such heterogeneous data are also presented in this book.

The next part of the book presents various data analytics models and their performance. Different big data techniques like association rule learning, Classification tree analysis, genetic algorithm, and machine learning are discussed with use cases. There are various parameters i.e. environmental factors, mobility, patient health history, etc., that can impact on spread rate. The categorization of these parameters is also discussed in this part of the book. The population with already existing diseases are more prone to COVID-19 and in the sequel the discussion of the vulnerable population is also discussed in the scope of this book.

The last section of the book presents a brief of global scenario affecting China, Italy, and the United States, as examples. Issues and challenges of data analytics regarding pandemics like COVID-19 are also presented with mitigation strategies that can be implemented. Recommendations for citizens, patients, and healthcare professionals are also suggested to overcome COVID-19. Finally, this book concludes with the open research and practical issues of COVID-19 control and future outlook to minimize the spread rate of COVID-19.

The main characteristics of this book are:

- A concise and summarized description of all topics.
- This book covers the recent pandemic of COVID-19 and presents ML models for predictions.
- Analytical models are explained with use case and scenario-based descriptions. This unique approach will certainly help readers to a better understanding of COVID-19.
- Issues, challenges, mitigation strategies, and recommendations are presented in simple terms that can be understood by a layman to better educate the public.
- Overall, in this book, analytical strategies of predictions for COVID-19 are explained in simple and easy terms so that it can be useful to a wide range of stakeholders, e.g. a layman to educate researchers, villages to metros and at the national to global levels.

The book is useful for undergraduates, postgraduates, industry researchers, and research scholars in the field of data analytics. It is also useful for the general public as recommendations to avoid widespread infections. We are sure that this book will be well received by all stakeholders.

ACKNOWLEDGMENT

We would like to thank many people who encouraged and helped us in various ways throughout the publication of this book, namely our colleagues, friends, and students. Special thanks to our family for their support and care.

We are thankful to the Honorable founder president of STES, Prof. M. N. Navale, founder secretary of STES, Dr. Mrs. S. M. Navale, Vice President (HR), Mr. Rohit M. Navale, Vice President (Admin), Ms. Rachana M. Navale, our Principal, Dr. A. V. Deshpande, Vice Principal, Dr. K. R. Borole, Dr. K. N. Honwadkar for their constant encouragement and inexplicable support.

We are also very much thankful to all our department colleagues at SKNCOE and Techno India College of Technology and for their continued support and help and for keeping us smiling all the time.

Last but not the least, our acknowledgments would remain incomplete if we do not thank the team of CRC Press who supported us throughout the development of this book. It has been a pleasure to work with the CRC Press team and we extend our special thanks to the entire team involved in the publication of this book.

Gitanjali R. Shinde
Asmita B. Kalamkar
Parikshit N. Mahalle
Nilanjan Dey

AUTHORS

Gitanjali R. Shinde has an overall experience of 11 years and is currently working as SPPU approved Assistant Professor in the Department of Computer Engineering, Smt. KashibaiNavale College of Engineering, Puno . She holds a PhD in Wireless Communication from CMI, Aalborg University, Copenhagen, Denmark, on Research Problem Statement "Cluster Framework for Internet of People, Things and Services" – her PhD was awarded on May 8, 2018. She obtained her ME (Computer Engineering) and BE (Computer Engineering) degrees from the University of Pune, Pune, in 2006 and 2012, respectively. She has received research funding for the project titled "Lightweight group authentication for IoT" by SPPU, Pune. She has presented a research article in the World Wireless Research Forum (WWRF) meeting, Beijing China. She has published 40+ papers in national and international conferences and journals. She is author of 3 books and is the editor of the book *The Internet of Everything: Advances, Challenges and application*, De Gruyter Press.

Asmita B. Kalamkar has 5 years of experience, and is currently working as SPPU approved Assistant Professor in the Department of Computer Engineering, Smt. KashibaiNavale College of Engineering, Pune. She obtained her BE (Computer Engineering) degree, 2013, and her ME (Computer Engineering) degree from SavitribaiPhule Pune University, Pune, 2015. She has published 10+ papers in national and international conferences and journals. She is the author of a book.

Parikshit N. Mahalle obtained his BE in Computer Science and Engineering from SantGadge Baba Amravati University, Amravati,

India, and ME in Computer Engineering from SavitribaiPhule Pune University, Pune, India. He completed his PhD in Computer Science and Engineering with a specialization in Wireless Communication from Aalborg University, Aalborg, Denmark. He was a post-doc Researcher at CMI, Aalborg University, Copenhagen, Denmark. Currently, he is working as Professor and Head of the Department of Computer Engineering at STES's Smt. KashibaiNavale College of Engineering, Pune, India. He has more than 20 years of teaching and research experience. He is serving as a subject expert in Computer Engineering, Research and Recognition Committee at several universities like SPPU (Pune) and SGBU (Amravati).He is a senior member of the IEEE, ACM member, Life member CSI, and Life member ISTE. Also, he is a member of the IEEE transaction on Information Forensics and Security, *IEEE Internet of Things Journal*. He is a reviewer for IGI Global – *International Journal of Rough Sets and Data Analysis (IJRSDA)*, Associate Editor for IGI Global - *International Journal of Synthetic Emotions (IJSE)* and *Inderscience International Journal of Grid and Utility Computing (IJGUC)*. He is a Member-Editorial Review Board for IGI Global – *International Journal of Ambient Computing and Intelligence (IJACI)*. He is also working as an Associate Editor for IGI Global – *International Journal of Synthetic Emotions (IJSE)*. He has also remained a technical program committee member for International conferences and symposia like IEEE ICC, IEEE INDICON, IEEE GCWSN, and IEEE ICCUBEA.

He is a reviewer for the *Springer Journal of Wireless Personal Communications*, reviewer for the *Elsevier Journal of Applied Computing and Informatics*, member of the Editorial Review Board of IGI Global – *International Journal of Ambient Computing and Intelligence (IJACI)*, member of the Editorial Review Board for the *Journal of Global Research in Computer Science*.

He has published more than 150 research publications with more than 1149 citations and H index 14. He has 5 edited books to his credit by Springer and CRC Press. He has 7 patents to his credit. He has also delivered invited talk on "Identity Management in IoT" to Symantec Research Lab, Mountain View, California. He has delivered more than 100 lectures at the national and international level on IoT, Big Data, and Digitization. He has authored 11 books on subjects like *Context-aware Pervasive Systems and Application* (Springer Nature Press), *Design and Analysis of Algorithms* (Cambridge University), *Identity Management for the Internet of Things* (River Publications), *Data*

Structure and Algorithms (Cengage Publications), and *Programming using Python* – (Tech-Neo Publications MSBTE). He had worked as Chairman of Board of Studies (Information Technology), SPPU, Pune. He is working as Member – Board of Studies (Computer Engineering), SPPU, Pune. He has been a member of the Board of Studies at several institutions like VIT (Pune), Govt. College (Karad), Sandeep University (Nashik), Vishwakarma University (Pune), and Dr. D. Y. Patil International University (Pune). He has also remained a technical program committee member for many International conferences.

He is a recognized PhD guide of SSPU, Pune, and is guiding 7 PhD students in the area of IoT and Machine Learning. Recently, 2 students have successfully defended their PhD He is also the recipient of the "Best Faculty Award" by Sinhgad Institutes and Cognizant Technology Solutions. His recent research interests include Algorithms, Internet of Things, Identity Management, and Security. He has visited a few countries like Denmark, France, Sweden, Germany, Austria, Norway, China, Switzerland, and Singapore.

Nilanjan Dey is an Assistant Professor in the Department of Information Technology at Techno India College of Technology, Kolkata, India. He is a Visiting Fellow of the University of Reading, UK. He was an honorary Visiting Scientist at Global Biomedical Technologies Inc., CA, USA (2012–2015). He was awarded his PhD from Jadavpur University in 2015. He has authored/edited more than 75 books with Elsevier, Wiley, CRC Press, and Springer, and published more than 300 papers. He is the Editor-in-Chief of the *International Journal of Ambient* Computing *and Intelligence*, IGI Global, and Associate Editor of IEEE Access and the *International Journal of Information Technology*, Springer. He is the Series Co-Editor of *Springer Tracts in Nature-Inspired Computing*, Springer Nature; Series Co-Editor of *Advances in Ubiquitous Sensing Applications for Healthcare*, Elsevier; Series Editor of *Computational Intelligence in Engineering Problem Solving and Intelligent Signal Processing and Data Analysis*; CRC. His main research interests include medical imaging, machine learning, computer-aided diagnosis, data mining, etc. He is the Indian Ambassador of the International Federation for Information Processing (IFIP) – Young ICT Group.

COVID-19 OUTBREAK

1.1 INTRODUCTION

The key to understanding a pandemic starts with an understanding of the disease itself and the progression of the natural course of the disease. The word "disease" is defined as the state that negatively affects the body of a living person, plant, or animal. A disease affects the body because of a pathogenic infection. The natural course of the disease starts before the onset of the infection, after which it progresses through the pre-symptomatic stage. The last stage is the clinical phase. In the clinical phase, a patient receives the prognosis of the disease. After successful treatment of the disease, the patient enters into the remission stage. Remission refers to a decrease in the symptoms or a complete disappearance of the disease. The patient needs to strictly follow instructions given by the doctor during the remission stage. This will ensure that the disease does not recur. If treatment is not successful, the patient can die or be chronically disabled. The following are some important terms that are used to represent the disease state:

(i) Case-fatality rate: It is defined as the ratio of the number of patients who die due to the disease to the number of people affected by it.
(ii) Observed survival rate: It is the prediction of the probability of survival.
(iii) Relative survival rate: It is defined as the percentage of the observed survival to the survival rate expectation.

Diseases are mainly categorized into two types:

(i) Congenital diseases
(ii) Acquired diseases

Congenital diseases exist in the body right from birth. These diseases are generally activated through genetic disorders, environmental factors, or a combination of both. These diseases are generally hereditary, i.e. passed on through generations, for example, hearing conditions and Down syndrome. In contrast to the former, acquired diseases spread through living organisms. These are not hereditary.

The acquired disease category is further classified into two types:

(i) Infectious diseases
(ii) Non-infectious diseases

Infectious diseases are induced by pathogens or viruses. They are also called communicable diseases. As the name suggests, these diseases are infectious. It means that if one person has contracted the infectious disease then the disease can be passed on to another person through air, food, water, touch (physical contact), etc. SARS and SARS COVID-19 are examples of infectious diseases.

Similarly, as the name suggests, non-infectious diseases do not occur due to any kind of infection. It means that a person with a non-infectious disease will not be able to spread the disease to a healthy person. Diseases such as cancer and auto-immune disorders are examples of non-infectious diseases.

Infectious disease can affect a healthy person in two ways.

(i) Direct transmission
(ii) Indirect transmission

When the pathogens travel from a patient to a healthy person without any middle carrier, then the transmission is referred to as direct transmission. Direct transmission can happen in the following ways:

• Coming in contact with the infected person.
• Via droplet infection (coughing, sneezing, and spitting).
• Coming in contact with the soil.

Animal bites are also one of the causes of direct transmission.

Whenever there is a reservoir of infection that can transmit the disease from a patient to a healthy person with a middle agent, then that transmission is known as indirect transmission. Indirect transmission can happen in the following ways.

- If pathogens are transmitted through food, water, etc., it is known as vehicle-borne disease.
- If pathogens are transmitted through the air, then it is known as airborne disease.
- If pathogens are transmitted through contaminated items like clothing, utensils, books, etc., it is known as fomite-borne disease.

After the diagnosis of the disease comes the most important part: the treatment. Treatment generally consists of targeting the biochemical reactions occurring due to pathogens. There are two ways to stop that reaction so that the infection will not spread:

(i) Prevention
(ii) Cure

Through prevention, symptoms of the infection can be reduced using painkillers so that patients can be at ease. Preventive measures also include immunization and vaccination. Through cure, particular drugs are used to kill the pathogen [1].

1.2 EPIDEMIC AND PANDEMIC OVERVIEW

1.2.1 Stages of Disease

Before studying the latest pandemic, it is very important to study basic terminologies associated with the pattern of disease spread. A diagrammatical overview of stages of the disease is depicted in Figure 1.1.

(i) **Sporadic**
When the occurrence of the disease is not regular and is infrequent, it is termed as sporadic.
(ii) **Endemic**
When the presence of the disease is constant in a particular geographical area, it is known as endemic. Endemic turns into a hyperendemic situation when a high level of disease occurrence is observed.
(iii) **Epidemic**
When there is a sudden rise in the number of patients with the same disease and within a particular area, it is termed as an epidemic.

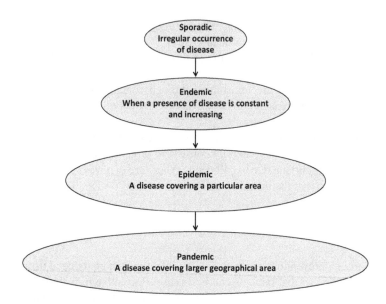

Figure 1.1   Stages of the disease.

(iv) **Pandemic**

   When epidemics affect larger geographical areas (including multiple countries and continents), it is known as a pandemic.

A disease takes the form of an epidemic when the following two conditions are met. First is when several people are affected by an illness/disease that has a similar nature of the disease and the same root cause, and the second is when the number of infected people rapidly increase over a period. When the epidemic crosses local boundaries and covers a wide geological area at the same time, it becomes a pandemic. A disease is listed under the category of pandemic because of its infectious nature. A pandemic does not give any information about the severity and impact of the disease. It merely states the fact that people across a wide geographical area are being infected with the disease.

   One more term that is majorly used while studying infectious diseases is "outbreak." Outbreak happens when a sudden rise in the number of patients is observed. Outbreaks can last a few days, weeks, or months. A pandemic is also sometimes referred to as an outbreak.

1.2.2 Pandemic Phases

When the World Health Organization (WHO) declares a pandemic alert for a disease, it follows six different phases.

- **Phase 1**: A pathogen/virus that exists in animals has not caused any kind of infection to humans.
- **Phase 2**: A pathogen/virus has infected humans.
- **Phase 3**: Small groups of people or random persons are infected with the virus.
- **Phase 4**: Human to human transmission is observed due to the outbreak at the community level.
- **Phase 5**: The disease has spread in multiple WHO regions.
- **Phase 6**: There is an outbreak of the disease in one or more regions different from the ones enlisted in Phase 5 [2].

1.2.2.1 Pandemic Risk Factors

A combination of spread risk and spark risk plays a primary role in pandemic risks. The spark risk occurs due to the transmission of the pathogen from animals to humans. These animals can be domestic animals or wild animals. The spread of the disease due to domestic animals is generally confined to densely populated areas. The key drivers of spark risks are live animal markets, wildlife reservoirs, etc. [3,4]. The spark risk is usually followed by the spread risk. As the name suggests, it concerns the transmission of the virus along with the genetic adaptation of the virus. The spread risk is influenced by the density of the population in the area, trade pattern, and travel pattern of the population [5].

1.2.2.2 Pandemic Mitigation

The most vital thing you can do in a pandemic is to be prepared for what's coming and be ready with response teams. These preparations can be categorized into the following categories:

(i) Pre-pandemic period
(ii) Spark period
(iii) Spread period

The pre-pandemic period, as the name suggests, is the stage before the pandemic. In this stage, continuous planning, simulation exercises, public health training, situational awareness, etc., are covered.

The spark period is defined as the detection of the initial outbreak of the pandemic. In this stage, laboratory confirmation of the pathogen, contact tracing, quarantine, situational awareness, etc., are covered.

The spread period is when the WHO globally declares the disease as a pandemic. In this stage, along with tracing and quarantine, vaccine or antiviral administration takes place. Treatment and care of patients is an important part of these three stages. While the vaccine is developed, there should be close coordination between the public and private sectors [6,7].

1.2.2.3 Situational Awareness

Situational awareness is having up-to-date information about potential infectious diseases and also knowing how to manage that threat with the available resources. Situational awareness is a key activity in the spark period as well as in the spread period. The support from healthcare facilities, media, and diagnostic facilities is very important. In this stage, it is important to understand the progression of pathogens and assemble all the necessary means to stop the spread. Because of the outbreak, the number of patients can increase within a short period. This sudden clinical surge should be efficiently managed [8].

1.2.2.4 History of Pandemics

Some pandemics stand out in history because of the catastrophe they have caused. We will study them in three parts. The first part includes notable pandemics before 1800, the second part covers notable pandemics in 1900, and the last part includes pandemics after 2000.

The first and one of the worst pandemics witnessed by the world was in 1347 named the Bubonic plague, also known as the Black Death pandemic [9]. In the wave of this pandemic, millions of people lost their lives. In the early 1500 the world witnessed the smallpox pandemic. The mortality rate was only 50% in some of the communities. This pandemic destroyed many native societies [10,11]. In 1881 the Fifth cholera pandemic occurred. More than 1.5 million deaths were reported [12]. The statistics are shown with the help of a graph in Figure 1.2 (a). From the graph, it is visible that Black Death was one of the worst pandemics witnessed by the world.

In the early 1900, the Spanish flu influenza pandemic occurred. Twenty to hundred million deaths were reported [13]. In 1950 the Asian flu influenza happened. A total of 1.5 million deaths were reported [14]. In 1968 the Hong Kong flu influenza pandemic occurred. A total of 1 million deaths were reported [15]. Finally in 1981, the HIV/AIDS pandemic occurred which claimed 36.7 million deaths. These pandemics caused a major economy loss [16]. The statistics are shown with the help of a graph in Figure 1.2 (b).

In the 2000s there was a whole new wave of pandemics. Severe acute respiratory syndrome (SARS) and the Middle East respiratory syndrome (MERS) were viral diseases. SARS occurred in 2003 which claimed 744 lives [17]. MERS occurred in 2012 which claimed 659 deaths [18]. In 2009 there was the Swine flu influenza pandemic. It was also known as H1N1. This virus claimed 575,500 lives all over the world [19]. In 2013 the West Africa Ebola virus pandemic caused 11,323 deaths [20]. The statistics are shown with the help of a graph in Figure 1.2(c).

From all the figures it is observed that these pandemics are a grave threat to humanity. The most recent pandemic is the Coronavirus pandemic (COVID-19). COVID-19 had been declared a pandemic in January 2020 by the World Health Organization (WHO). In a very short period, this pandemic has covered a large geographical area.

1.3 NOVEL CORONAVIRUS

The word "novel" means unknown or dealing with something new. From the beginning of the outbreak, extensive efforts are being taken by scientists and professionals all over the world. These extensive efforts include identification of the source of COVID-19, transmission pattern of the virus/pathogen, risk factors, disease progression, healthcare management, etc.

COVID-19 has a zoonotic origin. It means this virus was transmitted from animals to humans. Wuhan, China was the first city to experience the outbreak of this virus. It is considered that bats are the source of COVID-19. However, the main animal source behind COVID-19 has not been identified as of today. Also, the identification of the middle agent has not been done until now. In theory, the middle agent can be responsible for the spread of the virus from animals to humans. However, early detection of the cases suggests that most of the infected patients have acquired the disease from Wuhan; many of the patients were either working or visiting the city. As the number of patients began to increase, it was clear that a significant amount of human to human transmission was taking place. To contain the virus, Wuhan implemented comprehensive control measures which included

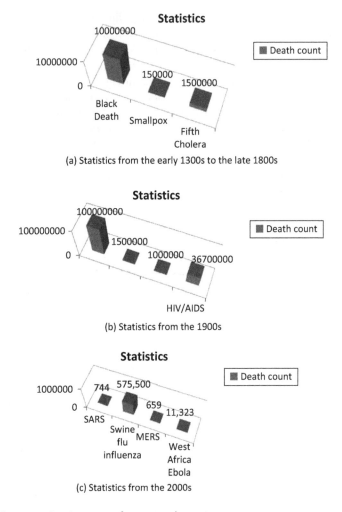

(a) Statistics from the early 1300s to the late 1800s

(b) Statistics from the 1900s

(c) Statistics from the 2000s

Figure 1.2 Statistics of past pandemics.

a complete lockdown of the city. Because of the status of Wuhan city as a transport hub and the mass movement of the population due to the Chinese New Year (*chunyun*), the infection quickly affected the mass population. The infected count was higher in the city of Wuhan, also with the highest traffic. When the situation started to take a disastrous route, Wuhan implemented strict measures to control the spread of the virus. These measures included the identification of patients

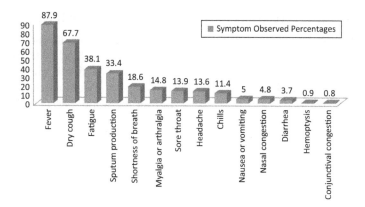

Figure 1.3 Symptoms observed in COVID-19 patients.

and their contacts and putting them under quarantine. Extreme social distancing was applied throughout the city to break human to human transmission. To date, most of the cases that are identified, one way or other, have a connection to Wuhan. The main objective behind imposing such strict measures was to stop community transmission.

Symptoms of COVID-19 range from a person showing no signs (asymptomatic) to a person having a severe case of pneumonia. Observed signs and symptoms of COVID-19 are as follows: fever, dry cough, fatigue, production of sputum, breathlessness, itchy throat, headache, myalgia or arthralgia, chills, vomiting, nasal blockage, loose motion, hemoptysis, and conjunctival congestion. As the number of symptoms and signs are overwhelming, the observed percentage associated with each sign is different [21]. The statistics are shown with the help of a graph in Figure 1.3.

It is clear from Figure 1.3 that most of the people are experiencing mild respiratory symptoms along with fever. These symptoms are observed after five to six days after the infection. It means that the incubation period for the virus is between two and fourteen days.

Infected patients have been categorized into the following three sections:

(i)   Patients experiencing mild to moderate symptoms
(ii) Patients experiencing severe symptoms
(iii) Patients in critical condition (failure of the respiratory system, septic shock, and multiorgan dysfunction/failure)

1.4 MEDICAL OVERVIEW – NATURE AND SPREAD

The COVID-19 outbreak was an unprecedented situation that no one saw it coming. As stated earlier, the origin of the COVID-19 outbreak was Wuhan. But still, the source of the infection is missing [22]. The situation around COVID-19 is rapidly becoming chaotic as the number of patients is rising all over the world. Not only the infected but the deceased count is increasing exponentially as well. Countries are applying the best possible control measures to curb the spread. But the count of patients is still increasing. Hence it is important to identify the reason behind the rising patient count. It is necessary to identify cases that became infected before a lockdown, the cases increased due to community transmission, the cases infected due to coming in contact with the hospital, or patients who acquired the infection from one of the infected family members. This study will help in the identification of asymptomatic carriers of the disease.

Human to human transmission of COVID-19 is confirmed but the transmission pattern and pathogenesis spread in humans is still a mystery [23,24]. It is also a big question that whether the pathogenesis of the virus is increased or decreased over time. If the transmission rate decreases, then eventually the spread of the disease will stop, and the outbreak will come to an end. If the transmission rate continues to rise, then the community outbreak will go beyond the point of management. As some patients have mild to no symptoms, it is becoming very difficult to identify them. If the study of asymptomatic infected cases is done, then the study can show how the antibodies present in the body are handling the viral load. It will also be helpful in the understanding of late symptom occurrence in asymptomatic patients. Asymptomatic infection can be very fatal in the case of children [25].

The WHO has confirmed that COVID-19 can spread through air droplets. If the droplet produced by the infected patient is inhaled by a healthy person, then the healthy person can contract the infection. There is also a feco-oral route of transmission, but this transmission route is declined in the WHO-China joint commission report. Still, contamination through human waste, infected water, and air conditioners can pose as viable threats [26]. Several patients infected with COVID-10 can have long-term neural, respiratory, and hepatic complications. These complications can lead to a very critical as well as fatal situation [27]. To date, we do not have a vaccine or a definite course of treatment for COVID-19. However, screening of new drug molecules can be beneficial in the course of treatment of COVID-19.

It has been observed that there are some recorded deaths of young people who after getting affected quickly succumbed to death. A detailed study on the subject will be able to reveal the genetic mutation that caused this fatality.

All over the world, many countries are facing this pandemic. Some of the countries have little success in controlling the COVID-19 situation. But still, there are numerous mysteries around the disease starting from the origin itself. This is an unprecedented situation. In this situation professionals from various disciplines need to work together to find a solution.

1.5 VULNERABILITY INDEX

COVID-19 is a fatal respiratory disease declared as a pandemic by the WHO. Because of the outbreak and quick spread of the disease, the information related to the disease is very limited. However, one observation was made: the group of patients with pre-existing medical conditions have high mortality rates.

Along with the previously mentioned group, patients who are very old, weak and with more than one chronic condition are also at a higher risk of having severe complications. The risk analysis of death is a little difficult, but a small study was conducted in Wuhan which shows the statistics, which is shown in Figure 1.4.

From the graph, it is seen that the analysis has classified deaths into four main groups:

Patients with cancer, high BP, and other chronic diseases: The percentage of deaths observed in this group was 6%.

Patients with diabetes: The percentage of deaths observed in this group was 7%.

Patients with heart diseases: The percentage of deaths observed in this group was 10%.

People aged 80 plus: The percentage of deaths observed in this group was the maximum at 15%.

One more observation concluded from the study is that patients with the same chronic condition might not experience the same symptoms [28]. Simple rules fail to apply in this situation; data analytics can play a major role here. However, data available in repositories or on

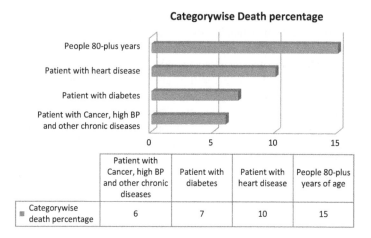

Categorywise Death percentage

	Patient with Cancer, high BP and other chronic diseases	Patient with diabetes	Patient with heart disease	People 80-plus years of age
■ Categorywise death percentage	6	7	10	15

Figure 1.4   Analysis of death groups.

social media are not in a format that can be used readily for data analysis. There are various challenges in using these data sources which is discussed in the next chapter. Moreover, various data storage services and data analytic techniques are also discussed in the subsequent chapters.

REFERENCES

1. Reynolds, T.A., Sawe, H.R., Rubiano, A.A., Shin, S.D., Wallis, L., and Mock, C.N. 2017. Strengthening Health Systems to Provide Emergency Care. In: Jamison, D.T., Gelband, H., Horton, S., Jha, P., Laxminarayan, R., Mock, C.N., and Nugent, R. (Eds.), *Disease Control Priorities: Improving Health and Reducing Poverty, 3rd Edition, Volume 9.*
2. World Health Organization. Online Available on. https://www.who .int/emergencies/diseases/novel-coronavirus-2019/.
3. Gilbert, M., Golding, N., Zhou, H., Wint, G.R.W., Robinson, T.P., et al. 2014. Predicting the Risk of Avian Influenza A H7N9 Infection in Live-Poultry Markets across Asia. *Nature Communications* 5(May): 1–7.
4. Jones, K.E., Patel, N.G., Levy, M.A., Storeygard, A., Balk, D., et al. 2008. Global Trends in Emerging Infectious Diseases. *Nature* 451(7181): 990–993.
5. Sands, P., Turabi, A.E.l., Saynisch, P.A., Dzau, V.J. 2016. Assessment of Economic Vulnerability to Infectious Disease Crises. *The Lancet* 388(10058): 2443–2448.

6. Brattberg, E., Rhinard, M. 2011. Multilevel Governance and Complex Threats: The Case of Pandemic Preparedness in the European Union and the United States. *Global Health Governance* 5(1): 1–21.
7. Hooghe, L., Marks, G. 2003. Unraveling the Central State, but How? Types of Multi-Level Governance. *American Political Science Review* 97(2): 233–243.
8. ASPR (Assistant Secretary for Preparedness and Response). 2014. Public Health and Medical Situational Awareness Strategy. Strategy Document for Situational Awareness Implementation Plan. Washington, DC: U.S. Department of Health and Human Services.
9. DeWitte, S.N. 2014. Mortality Risk and Survival in the Aftermath of the Medieval Black Death. *PLoS One* 9(5): e96513.
10. Jones, D.S. 2006. The Persistence American Indian Health Disparities. *American Journal of Public Health* 96(12): 2122–2134.
11. Diamond, J. 2009. *Guns, Germs, and Steel: The Fates of Human Societies*. New York: Norton.
12. Chisholm, H. 1911. Cholera. *Encyclopedia Britannica* 11(6): 265–266.
13. Johnson, N.P.A.S., Mueller, J. 2002. Updating the Accounts: Global Mortality of the 1918–1920 'Spanish' Influenza Pandemic. *Bulletin of the History of Medicine* 76(1): 105–115.
14. Viboud, C., Simonsen, L., Fuentes, R., Flores, J., Miller, M.A., Chowell, G. 2016. Global Mortality Impact of the 1957–1959 Influenza Pandemic. *The Journal of Infectious Diseases* 212(11): 738–745.
15. Mathews, J.D., Chesson, J.M., McCaw, J.M., McVernon, J. 2009. Understanding Influenza Transmission, Immunity, and Pandemic Threats. *Influenza and Other Respiratory Viruses* 3(4): 143–149.
16. World Health Organization (WHO). *Global Health Observatory (GHO) Data*. http://www.who.int/gho/hiv/en [Accessed: 25-April-2020].
17. Wang, M.D., Jolly, A.M. 2004. Changing Virulence of the SARS Virus: The Epidemiological Evidence. *Bulletin of the World Health Organization* 82(7): 547–548.
18. Arabi, Y.M., Balkhy, H.H., Hayden, F.G., Bouchama, A., Luke, T., et al. 2017. Middle East Respiratory Syndrome. *New England Journal of Medicine* 376(6): 584–594.
19. Dawood, F.S., Iuliano, A.D., Reed, C., Meltzer, M.I., Shay, D.K., et al. 2012. Estimated Global Mortality Associated with the First 12 Months of 2009 Pandemic Influenza A H1N1 Virus Circulation: A Modelling Study. *The Lancet Infectious Diseases* 12(9): 687–695.

20. WHO (World Health Organization). 2016a, April 15. *Ebola Situation Report*. Weekly data report,
21. Report of the WHO-China Joint Mission on Coronavirus Disease 2019 (COVID-19) [Pdf]. World Health Organization, February 28, 2020.
22. Singhal, T. 2020. A Review of Coronavirus Disease-2019 (COVID-19). *Indian Journal of Pediatrics* 87(4): 281–286.
23. Rothe, C., Schunk, M., Sothmann, P., Bretzel, G., Froeschl, G., et al. 2020 Machr 5. Transmission of 2019-nCoV Infection from an Asymptomatic Contact in Germany. *The New England of Medicine* 382(10): 970–971.
24. Chan, J.F.W., Yuan, S., Kok, K.H., To, K.K.W., Chu, H., et al. 2020. A Familial Cluster of Pneumonia Associated with the 2019 Novel Coronavirus Indicating Person-to-Person Transmission: A Study of a Family Cluster. *The Lancet* 395(10223): 514–523, 2.
25. Xiaoxia, L., Liqiong, Z., Hui, D., Jingjing, Z., Yuan, L., et al. 2020. SARS-CoV-2 Infection in Children. *The New England Journal of Medicine*. doi:10.1056/NEJMc2005073.
26. Moriarty, L.F., Plucinski, M.M., Marston, B.J., Kurbatova, E.V., Knust, B., et al. 2020. Public Health Responses to COVID-19 Outbreaks on Cruise Ships-Worldwide, February-March 2020. *MMWR Morbidity and Mortality Weekly Report* 69(12): 347–352.
27. Beth, Russell, Charlotte, Moss, Anne, Rigg, Claire, Hopkins, Sophie, Papa. 2020. Van HemelrijckMieke and Ageusia Are Emerging as Symptoms in Patients with COVID-19: What Does the Current Evidence Say? *Ecancer* 14: ed98.
28. Page, Michael Le. 2020, 11 March. Why Is It so Hard to Calculate How Many People Will Die from Covid-19? *New Scientist*. www.newscientist.com/article/mg24532733-700-why-is-it-sohard-to-calculate-how-many-people-will-die-from-covid-19/.

DATA PROCESSING AND KNOWLEDGE EXTRACTION

2.1 DATA SOURCES AND RELATED CHALLENGES

Prediction of the mortality and spread rate plays a very important role in the control measures for pandemic diseases like COVID-19. Based on this prediction, precautionary measures can be taken by public, government, and healthcare systems [1,2]. These predictions are also helpful to pharmaceutical companies for formulating and manufacturing drugs at a faster rate. There are various techniques and models to forecast the spread/mortality rate. This forecasting is done based on the data that is available for the prediction. In the case of pandemic diseases, researchers refer data from various data sources and use different models for data analysis. The data can be referred from the following data sources [3–8]:

- World Health Organization
- National repositories
- Online social media
- Mobile phone data
- News websites

The authenticity of the data source is debatable as these data sources are not endorsed by any standardization authority/agency; however, most of these data sources are nationalized repositories and WHO repositories. Data from online social media and news websites may be in different formats, as different data sources may store data in different forms. Few data may be in structured format while others may be in an unstructured or semi-structured format. This heterogeneity of data is a major issue in data analysis. Analysis of various data sources and prediction techniques can be useful for model selection [9]. Various sources of data, their challenges, and various potential online storage service providers are shown in Figure 2.1.

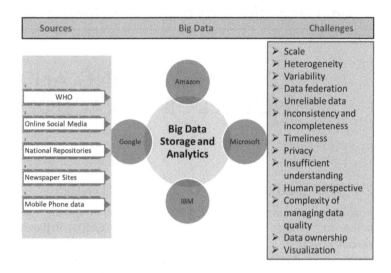

Figure 2.1   Big Data sources, challenges and service providers.

There are various challenges in big data and these are well explained in the literature [10–15]. This section discusses the challenges related to COVID-19 datasets.

- Scale: Considering the size of the data in the case of COVID-19, we face two exactly opposite scenarios. First, in the initial period of the pandemic, the data available is not in big volume; hence, statistical analysis or training AI models is very difficult. Forecasting may be incorrect as less data is available for training the model. In the second case, after a few days have gone and the spread has increased, more data might be available, and researchers may find a few more parameters important for forecasting. The prediction of COVID-19 is not only dependent on the death and infection count, but it is also dependent on the mobility rate. Researchers have been trying to analyze the impact of environmental factors like temperature, air humidity, and wind speed on the spread rate of COVID-19. For such an analysis, international/local mobility data and metrological data are required. But this data is being generated every second and the size of that data might range in zettabytes or may be in Yottabytes as well. In the first case, training the AI/ML models on a small dataset; and in the second case, processing such high-volume data are the major challenges of forecasting mechanisms.

• Heterogeneity: As mentioned earlier, scientists are working to find out the correlation between the spread rate and various parameters like environmental factors, mobility, patient's age, gender, and medical history for the prediction of the COVID-19 death count in the near future. These data may be in different formats: few may be in text format, few may be in image format, and so on. As these data include weather reports, patient health reports, international/ national flights/train data, each follows different data formats for representation. Heterogeneity of data is again a major concern while retrieving knowledge from these data sources.

• Variability: COVID-19 has spread across most of the countries of the world; it is not limited to China where it was first detected. Information about infection count, death count, and names of the infected places have been made available worldwide and at the national level to make people aware of the spread. This data can be very helpful for statistical analysis. This data is stored and shared by various sources like news websites, online social media platforms, and mobile apps. Though data is homogeneous, there are variations in the formats used by sources sharing these data. Data processing of these data variations is a crucial task for data analytics.

• Data federation: As mentioned earlier, although data may be homogeneous, it is in heterogeneous formats due to the various sources that are sharing it. Furthermore, prediction techniques may require multi-feature data to integrate such heterogeneity and variable data is a major hurdle for forecasting.

• Unreliable data: Reliability of data often plays a crucial role in predictions not only in the healthcare domain but also in various fields like business, stock market, weather forecasting, etc. As various data sources are available to share data, and as they may not be endorsed by any standardization organization, trusting these data sources is difficult.

• Inconsistency and incompleteness: Forecasting is done based on specific parameters; however, in data processing it is possible that a few parameters may have missing values, i.e. the data may be incomplete. In such situations the analysis of data might result in poor prediction due to data loss. Statistical analysis or ML models have various techniques to address this issue; however, this may come at the cost of accuracy.

- Timeliness: High-volume data may need a longer time for data processing and, hence, for predictions as well. However, in many situations, predictions may be needed in a shorter time. There is a need to have a data storage format thereby minimizing the response time for a query. Data storage should have an indexing structure and other mechanisms to process such high-volume data with a faster response time.
- Privacy: Nowadays data is money; sharing data publicly may cost a lot to the individual/country. For the forecasting, a COVID-19 patient's sensitive information, i.e. health data, location, and other information, may be required for analysis. This information may be stored in repositories; the security of these data sources is of prime concern. In this situation, information about the infected locations in the country may also be shared with data repositories. Leakage of such information may result in serious consequences for a community.
- Insufficient understanding: As mentioned earlier, big data is heterogeneous and big in size; it has various formats and may be multidomain. Insufficient understanding of such a variety of data may lead to inaccurate predictions. Hence, understanding of such multidimensional data and domain knowledge as well as expertise is required for data analysis.
- Human perspective: Humans have the ability to think, which machines don't have. Although there are many advances in AI and ML, there is still no match to the human brain. Hence, in the forecasting mechanism there must be scope to add the human perspective for data analysis. Big data analysis techniques must take inputs from experts in the field for analyzing the data and predicting the output.
- The complexity of managing data quality: As discussed earlier, for prediction, multidomain data may be required and due to the various features of big data mentioned above, it may be very difficult to maintain data quality. Because of the various features, there is a need to have a strategy to overcome these hurdles and maintain the quality of the data. The quality of data is correlated to the prediction of spread rate/infection count.
- Data ownership: Data sources share data publicly; however, there is a concern of losing control over data. There must be a mechanism of sharing data without losing control. Organizations with big data are concerned with the issue of

data sharing; hence, there is a need to identify techniques to keep control over the data while sharing.

• Visualization: Though machine algorithms will work on these data, the visualization of data and the predictions should be in a format understandable to humans. Otherwise the user may get lost in the big data and would not be able to retrieve knowledge out of it. Visualization mechanisms are needed in a form that can give a clear picture about the knowledge that is retrieved from big data.

2.2 DATA STORAGE: PLATFORM

It is very difficult and costly for any individual organization to store big data locally for providing services to the user. Due to the problem of local storage the role of remote storage on the Internet, i.e. cloud computing, came into discussion. Cloud storage is used as Infrastructure as a Service (IaaS) where big data is not stored at any local machine; it is stored in the cloud by various service providers. There are various cloud service providers that are available to store big data and provide services to the end-users. Users can access these data through various APIs which are provided by cloud owners. Similarly, big data of COVID-19 can be placed on the cloud storage and the owner can access these data using APIs, and by this the issue of local storage of COVID-19 data can be resolved. Nowadays almost all organizations are using cloud platforms for data storage due to the requirement of decentralization. Users can access data from any location and using any machine. The quality of cloud service providers is based on various parameters, such as how much data can be stored, how fast data can be accessed, how many services are provided, and the security of data.

A few widely used big data analytics platforms are provided by potential IT leaders like Google, Amazon, Microsoft, and IBM. These cloud service providers provide various cloud services for big data storage, processing, and also for data analytics; it is termed as Big Data as a Service (BDaaS). Cloud services are also available for computation and database management. In this digital era, most of the data are generated because of the Internet of Things; cloud platforms also provide services for IoT. AI and ML models are mostly used for big data analytics, in view of these cloud platforms also provides AI and ML services. Organizations gain value out of data stored on the cloud, and keeping this data secure by providing secure access is an important functionality of storage platforms. To do so, the cloud platforms provide security, identity, and access services. Cloud platforms also provide various services like mobile and networking services. In this section cloud platforms of Google, Amazon, Microsoft, and IBM are discussed [16–18].

2.2.1 Storage Services

Various IT leaders have high volumes of data, and to store these data, big servers and software will be needed. Using cloud computing, the need of a dedicated infrastructure can be removed. Cloud computing provides various services, and among all these services, storage services are the basic features of cloud computing. Storage services provide mechanisms to store and handle heterogeneous as well as high volume data. The end user can access the data through various cloud applications. There are two types of storage provided by cloud, i.e. object storage and block storage.

- **Object Storage**

    In this type of storage, the unit of data storage is in object form. Object is the basic abstract and distinct entity of data in the repository [32]. Objects consist of various parts, i.e. actual data, metadata about data, and the unique address/identification of the object. This type of data is protected by keeping multiple copies of the object at various geographical places. In this digital world, data cannot be static with respect to the volume. Data can increase in volume; hence, in the object storage facility of data, growth is accommodated. A new node can be easily created for newly added data as scalability is an important feature of cloud computing.
- **Block Storage**

    In block storage, data is stored in a more standard format. Data is divided into same sized blocks, and these blocks are kept at separate places as separate entities. Here, file folder arrangement is not used to store blocks, and each block has a unique address for identification. The network of virtual storage areas deals with the logical management of blocks, which is provided by block storage services. In the virtual area storage, the user can mount data by using any operating system in the same way data is mounted on a physical disc. The smaller blocks of data are spread over the storage area which results in efficient storage management. Storage services provided by Amazon, Microsoft, Google, and IBM are discussed as follows.

• **Amazon S3**
  Amazon provides both ways of storage services, i.e. object and block storage. Amazon Web Services (AWS) Simple Storage Service (S3) is Amazon's object storage service. This service provides cost-effective and flexible storage of data. The word "bucket" is used as an abstraction of storage; in one bucket nearly 5 TB objects can reside, and S3 offers 99.99% availability of data for a year.
  Amazon S3 provides robust, scalable, and secure data storage for various use cases like big data analytics, AI and ML, and many more.
  Amazon S3 provides three different classes of storage to accommodate different use cases, i.e. in many applications data access may be required frequently, and in few cases data access may be required but not in higher frequency.

• Amazon S3 Standard: Amazon S3 standard class offers object storage for data which requires access in higher frequency. The data that needs to be accessed in higher frequency requires an efficient, robust, and higher availability platform, which is provided by Amazon S3 standard. This type of storage is suitable for mobile applications, websites, content distribution, game sites, and big data analytics applications due to its lower latency and higher throughput. In Amazon S3, policies are implemented for data object management and migrations of the storage class.

• Amazon S3 Standard – Infrequent Access (Standard – IA): Amazon Standard IA class provides storage service for applications in which data is not accessed frequently. Data can be accessed infrequently; however, faster access is required in such types of applications. Faster data access and higher throughput are provided at a low cost. This service is useful for backups, and application storage is needed for a longer period. Policies like transferring data objects in various storage classes without application change are required in such types of storage.

• Amazon Glacier:
  This is a secure storage service with lower pricing. The service provides reliable data storage irrespective of the volume of data, and provides three different access points based on the duration of access, i.e. short duration access, and long duration access.

Amazon also offers block storage called AWS Elastic Block Storage (EBS) with block sizes ranging from 4 GB to 16 TB. This service provides four volumes based on access time and volume of data.

* **Microsoft Azure Blob Storage**
  Microsoft's object store, i.e. Blob Storage, provides storage for unstructured data in the form of objects. In this storage, binary or different types of text data can be stored, i.e. data can be of various forms like audio files, video files, or document or application exe files. Two different types of storage classes are provided by Azure. These classes are cost-efficient as costing is based on data access frequency and these are discussed as follows.

* Azure Hot Storage:
  This type of storage is for data that requires a higher accessing frequency, such as the type of access with lower latency, higher throughput, and higher availability.

* Azure Cool Storage:
  Azure Cool Storage is for the data which is not accessed in higher frequency; however, it requires throughput similar to hot storage.

  Azure uses data replication to provide high data availability; data is replicated in two ways: it keeps the replica either at the same storage center or some other center. In this way data can be safe in case of hardware failure. As the replica is stored at other centers, data is safe irrespective of failure in the primary storage.

  Azure also provides block storage in two forms: Standard and Premium storage, for high volume data ranging from 1 GB to 4 TB; premium storage provides faster access than standard storage.

* **Google Cloud Storage Service**
  Like Amazon and Microsoft, Google also provides object storage service, i.e. Google Cloud Storage service. It provides high data availability, seamless data access, and secure storage with low pricing. It provides four categories of services, which are described as follows.

* Multiregional Storage: This type of storage is for data that requires higher frequency. Data is kept safe by keeping data objects at multiple storage centers. These centers (at least two) must be in geographically distinct regions so that the availability

of data can be improved. This type of storage can be used by organizations where data security and data availability are of prime importance.

- Regional Storage: This is a cost-effective data storage option where data objects are stored at regions; here, data availability can be the issue. This can be a storage solution for applications that require data storage at a lower cost.

- Nearline Storage: This type is useful for short duration storage, i.e. a few months. In this, the cost is lower than other categories of storage; however, data availability may be marginally lower. Applications where storage is required for short periods can use this type of storage.

- Coldline Storage: This type of object storage is used to store data that is not required in higher frequency. This storage can be useful for backups.

- Google also provides block storage for data volume ranging from 1 GB to 64 TB. It provides two categories of block storage. These storage types provide the highest input output per second for reading and writing data; it also provides maximum throughput.

- **IBM's Bluemix Cloud Object Storage Service**

  IBM offers object storage, i.e. Bluemix Cloud Object Storage service, where objects of smaller sizes up to 5 GB can be uploaded using an API. In this, the facility of automatically storing multiple objects in a single manifest file is provided. This manifest file can range up to 5 TB in size. Here, for data availability, data can be stored in multiple centers, in the same region, or in different regions, i.e. cross-regional data storage.

  IBM also provides four categories of storage as follows:

  - Standard Storage: This type of storage is used for data that is accessed in higher frequency.

  - Vault Storage: This type of storage is used for data that is not frequently accessed, and storage is required for a shorter period. It may be used for backup and archives.

  - Cold Vault Storage: This is also used for data that is not frequently accessed, and the storage duration is more than 90 days at a lower cost.

  - Flex Storage: This type of storage is used for data that requires dynamic access; however, the cost of such storage is higher than other storage services.

IBM also provides block storage service with smaller storage capacity than other cloud storage providers and for data that doesn't require higher access time.

2.2.2 Big Data Analytics Services

In this digital era, storage of data is not a big challenge as discussed above. Many leading companies are providing storage services at an affordable cost. Nowadays, retrieving knowledge out of this data is more challenging and important for revenue collection. In a pandemic like COVID-19, faster analysis is more important as it can save invaluable human life for which big data analytics services can be very useful. A few such big data analytics services provided by Amazon, Google, Microsoft, and IBM are discussed as follows.

a) **Amazon Elastic Search Service**

Amazon ES provides services to manage and analyze data with higher access time using open source APIs. It provides an easy way to create domains and provides higher throughput using indexing. It also provides visualization using Kibana 6.2 and REST clients which support the Amazon ES search. This is used widely in applications like live monitoring and analytics of log files as it supports various open source tools of data analytics. It is used by organizations like Claranet, Expedia, MirrorWeb, Graylink, and Wyng.

b) **Microsoft Azure HDInsight (Big Data Analytics Solution)**

Microsoft Azure HDInsight service provides an understandable and easy portal to deploy data on clusters using virtual machines. Here, users have the facility of creating a number of nodes inside the cluster for data analysis. The best part of this is that the user needs to pay only for the amount service used. It also provides support for cluster creation for Hadoop, Spark, Kafka, etc. It is used by organizations like LG CNS, ASOS, and Roche.

c) **Google Cloud Dataproc**

Google Cloud Dataproc provides faster, easier, automated, and organized cluster formation at lower cost. The best part of it is that the upscaling of clusters is done within 90 seconds. Every cluster is secured with encryption techniques and supports open source clusters like Apache Hadoop and Presto. Here, users need to pay for resources that are in use; the cost can be minimized by turning of clusters that are not in use. It is used by various organizations like Twitter, Pandora, and Metro.

d) **IBM Analytics Engine**

IBM's Analytics Engine provides data analytics services with open source platforms like Apache Hadoop and Spark. It provides the facility of storing data as object storage, and clusters can be created for data analysis when required instead of creating clusters permanently. This facility provides scalable and flexible platform data analytics.

2.2.3 Data Warehousing Services

Data warehouses store data from multiple sources and keep it online for user queries; hence, it requires efficient data storage. A data warehouse can store data of various categories like structured, unstructured, and semi-structured. Big data can be easily stored and accessed by data warehousing, and it also supports big data analysis. Data warehousing can be helpful in storing big data of COVID-19 on the cloud storage, and clients can easily access these data using APIs, by which the issue of COVID-19 data availability can be resolved. A few data warehousing services are discussed as follows.

a) **Amazon Redshift**

Amazon provides a cost-efficient, well-organized, and faster data warehousing service called Redshift. It provides data analysis using SQL and various tools of business intelligence with a higher response time of query processing and with guaranteed data protection. Organizations like Lyft, Pfizer (a pharmaceutical company), McDonald, FOX Corporation, NTT DOCOMO, many more use the Amazon Redshift.

b) **Azure SQL Data Warehouse**

Microsoft's Azure SQL Data Warehouse provides parallel execution of the query, which results in faster query processing. In this, the control node divides the query into subqueries that can be executed in parallel, and these subqueries are assigned to compute nodes. In this way, the response to queries is achieved in a faster time.

c) **Google BigQuery**

Google's BigQuery provides facilities for creating an ML model with the help of SQL. In this model, infrastructure support is not required and hence, there is no need for a database administrator. It is used by more than 500 companies such as UPS, American Eagle, eBay, HSBC, and Nielsen.

d) **IBM Db2 Warehouse on Cloud**

IBM's Db2 Warehouse provides in-memory processing of data, and data is in a columnar table format. This provides higher efficiency of query retrieval due to its compatibility with Oracle and Netezza. It is used by various companies like AMC Networks, City Furniture, and Constance Hotel.

Selection of an appropriate cloud platform for any application/organization is dependent on the type of data that needs to be stored, the frequency at which data can be accessed, the cost involved, level of security required for the data, open source tools provided for data storage/data analytics, and, most importantly, the availability of data.

2.3 DATA PROCESSING

In any application of data analysis, data may be taken from various sources as mentioned in the first section. Data may be taken from repositories, mobile phones, news websites, or online social media platforms. Data from such sources may follow different formats; however, for analyzing these data it should be in a uniform format. Data preparation is the important phase of data analysis and that includes data cleaning, data formatting, and converting data in a specific format [19,20]. In the case of COVID-19, data may not be in the form that can be directly used for data analysis. There may be incompleteness and impurities in the data. Hence the data of COVID-19 should also be first prepared and pre-processed/cleaned before data analysis. Data processing includes data cleaning as the initial and important step after data acquisition. The steps involved in data processing are depicted in Figure 2.2.

The quality and performance of the extracted knowledge depend on the design, performance of the method, as well as the quality of the underlying data. But data usually comes with redundancies, inconsistencies, and missing instances. Hence, the poorer the quality of the data, the poorer will be the knowledge extracted from it. Data preprocessing is one of the major tasks in the knowledge extraction process. A clean and complete dataset will be able to produce rich knowledge and rich conclusions.

The same data preprocessing approach used in data mining cannot be used to implement data preprocessing. As the size of the data increases, new approaches should be implemented.

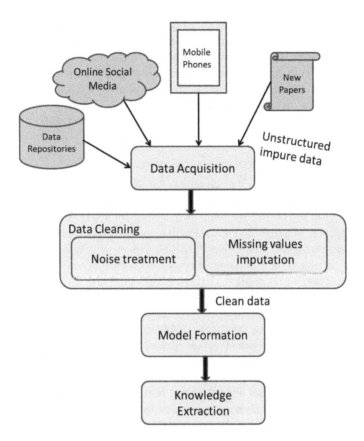

Figure 2.2 Data processing steps.

Data preprocessing techniques are implemented before the implementation of the data analysis technique. It is one of the important phases in the knowledge extraction process. Data cannot be directly taken for data analysis as it contains redundancies and inconsistencies. As days are passing, the size of data production is growing enormously. As the size of the data is huge, the analysis depends on the mechanisms used in data preprocessing. Data preprocessing is the ability to transform data according to the requirements. Data preprocessing is implemented in the early stages of classification and regression problems. Data preprocessing is not only used in data mining, but it is also used in the machine learning domain. Many researchers are now giving more attention to data preprocessing techniques in order to improve the efficiency and accuracy of the model.

Whenever we consider data mining techniques, the baseline assumption is that the dataset is complete or there is no noise in the data. But in real-time scenarios, the data is always incomplete and dirty. Data preprocessing techniques are implemented in order to remove the noise from the data or to fill the missing data [19].

2.3.1 Missing Values Imputation

A missing value is a value which was not recorded during the collection of data because of the incomplete sampling process, restrictions related to the cost of the data, or due to restrictions placed on data collection. In a real-time scenario, these missing values tend to create severe problems for developers. Dealing with missing values is one of the difficult tasks. If missing values are not handled properly, often it may create wrong results. These missing values also affect the efficiency of the extracted knowledge.

There are multiple methods available for handling the problem of missing values in the dataset. The first method is to completely eliminate those instances that contain the missing data. However, this approach is easy, but it creates a major bias in the output, as some of the vital instances can be deleted in the process. Using statistics, seminal work on data imputation has been designed. In this method, the model is created using probability functions. These probability functions are applied to the data considering the missing instances. The maximum likelihood function is used to fill in the missing values. This technique is widely used nowadays.

2.3.2 Noise Treatment

Whenever we are dealing with data mining algorithms, the base assumption is that the data has no disturbance. But in the real-time scenario, it is hardly the case because when data is collected from different sources, corruption in the data is always there. It becomes mandatory to deal with corruption/noise in the data because the quality of the data collected directly affects the results of data mining. If we consider supervised learning problems, then this noise can affect the selection of attributes along with its output. Sometimes both the input and the output are affected. If noise is present in the input, then it is also referred to as attribute noise. The worst case is observed when this noise affects the output. It means there is a considerable amount of bias in the output. This type of noise is usually studied under classification problems; it is referred to as class noise. In order to deal with the noise in the data, two methods are used. They are listed as follows:

(i) Data polishing
(ii) Noise filters

In the first method, the noise in the data is eliminated by data polishing if the labeling of the instance is compromised. Even partial data polishing can be beneficial, but this is a very tough task. It can be implemented in case of a small amount of data. In the second method, noisy data is eliminated in the training phase only.

The data after cleaning is converted into the format required for data analysis, and knowledge is retrieved from this data using various data analytics techniques.

2.4 KNOWLEDGE EXTRACTION

2.4.1 Knowledge Extraction Based on Data Types

There is a need for different types of knowledge extraction techniques for different types of data, i.e. text, audio, video, etc., as the structure of each data is different; hence, the same method cannot be applicable for all. In the case of COVID-19, data can be in text, audio, or image form, as these data are retrieved from various sources, discussed in the first section. There is a need for different techniques to retrieve knowledge from these heterogeneous data. In the literature, various methods are presented for knowledge extraction from different types of data [21–25].

2.4.1.1 Knowledge Extraction from Text Data

Text data is generally unstructured data. This unstructured data needs to be transformed into structured data through the annotation of semantic knowledge. Knowledge extraction systems can be classified into different categories as follows:

(i) Logical structures
(ii) Nature of data sources
(iii) Linguistic components
(iv) Domain criteria

Low-level structures in the text are categorized as follows:

(i)   Named entity recognition (NER)
(ii) Relation extraction (RE)
(iii) Event extraction (EE)

NER helps in finding out the related knowledge about the entities that are named. RE helps in the identification of the relationship between those named entities. Lastly, EE helps in the identification of the events in the text. In order to extract the most meaningful and relevant knowledge, various techniques are researched, i.e. natural language processing, machine learning, text mining and computational linguistics. Extraction approaches to extract knowledge are as follows:

(i)   Rule-based method: In this method, lexical patterns, syntactical patterns, and semantic constraints are used by NER to identify the existence of similar entities.
(ii) Learning-based method: In this method, machine learning is used to find out different entities along with their classification. Machine learning methods are further categorized into three sections as follows:
      a. Supervised learning
      b. Unsupervised learning
      c. Semi-supervised learning
         Supervised and unsupervised algorithms use a huge amount of training data in order to achieve high accuracy. In the case of semi-supervised algorithms, labeled as well as unlabeled data are used with a little bit of supervision.
(iii) Hybrid method: This method is a combination of two or more methods. These methods try to cut short efforts and achieve high accuracy. However, experts are needed to design and develop such methods.

Having a huge amount of unstructured data makes this task very challenging for KE. EE from the unstructured document is an even more challenging task. However, various techniques are designed to automatically give the labels to the data so that it can be used for training purposes. But this labeling method increases the noise because of missing or wrong labels. In this situation, deep learning and machine learning techniques are implemented. The only challenge is to identify what technique will be most efficient for the current problem.

In order to eliminate sequential extraction of knowledge from NER, RE hybrid neural network models and joint models have been designed. These models handle errors by splitting the NER and RE into two different but parallel tasks. Joint models combined with deep learning are proving to be most effective for feature extraction from unstructured documents. As the unstructured documents are complex and heterogeneous in nature, this job becomes more difficult. NLP tools and techniques are vital in the KE domain. NLP started with some base techniques like word segmentation, part of speech tagging, parsing, NER, and RE among entities and words, etc. Research on schema is divided into two categories. The first is to find out the universal schema; and the second, collaborative filtering. RE's focus is on discovering the relation between these entities. For this purpose, several supervised as well as unsupervised algorithms have been designed.

2.4.1.2 Knowledge Extraction from Image Data

Due to the sudden rise in social media use and globalization, the production of image data has increased. This type of data is visually very rich, but it is in a structured format. Extracting meaningful semantic and visual construct is one of the challenging tasks. In KE, image feature extraction, understanding of the scene, and text recognition are some very important areas to focus on. In order to find out objects in the given image, feature extraction can be helpful. Along with feature extraction, different classification and segmentation methods can be used for the same purpose. Feature extraction from an image can be done with the help of the Scale Invariant Feature Transform (SIFT). In this method text resides inside the image and this type of knowledge is generally very large. Text extraction methods are used in order to extract meaningful knowledge from the image. But this task comes with its own set of challenges--it is very difficult to find out the text due to different languages, sizes, orientation, contrast, background colors, etc. Various approaches have been designed for this purpose, but these approaches have limitations like domain or language. For the extraction of text from an image, no single technique is available that can be implemented in all scenarios. The benefits of KE from images are high accuracy and less complexity. However, if the image in question contains noise then that noise must be removed before the implementation of KE. To get a better understanding of the visual/ scene, a top-down, bottom-up, or combined approach is used. In real-time or dynamic scenarios, a full understanding of the scene and the static and dynamic occlusions makes KE very challenging.

2.4.1.3 Knowledge Extraction from Audio Data

Nowadays, call centers, music fields, and podcasting are the major players which generate a huge amount of audio data. Audio data contains knowledge that is different from image or video data. The type of knowledge that can be extracted from audio data can be very helpful in predictive and descriptive analytics in big data. For speech to text conversion, Automatic Speech Recognition is widely used. However, for more accurate results, hybrid feature extraction is used. For event detection purposes, a combination of Support Vector Machine (SVM) and Artificial Neural Network (ANN) techniques are used. Some events such as the use of musical instruments like drum, hammering, and the voice of laughter are very difficult to handle even while using the above-mentioned techniques. Sound or event extraction transforms audio notes into descriptions using symbols. If only mono channel audio is needed, then it is achieved using long- or short-term memory recurrent neural networks. In this technique, overlapping voices are completely ignored. Multiple low- and high-level features can be extracted from audio data. The mid-level features are used in the implementation of applications such as automatic music generators, mash-up formations, etc. The conversion of a letter to sound is also possible in KE audio. This can be implemented in languages like Amharic, Hindi, and Tamil. This is a very challenging field, facing challenges such as understanding speech in various languages and higher frequency, overlapping sound, etc. Analysis of arbitrary soundtracks along with timestamp occurrence of music is achieved using semantic KE. Semantic KE is used to extract music and text knowledge with the help of segmentation and classification. An integrated approach of speech detection and verification can be very useful in speech recognition and speech analysis.

2.4.1.4 Knowledge Extraction from Video Data

Video KE is facing its own set of challenges such as differentiation in background and foreground, speech-to-text and text-to-speech transformations, labeling automation, and extraction of text from video feeds. Different semantic labels are provided using semantic detection at various levels. Retrieval of high dimensional features along with annotation combination is a very popular area of research. In this area, different projections along with data generalizations and reduction techniques are implemented in order to eliminate wrong results. Temporal KE is used to extract some common features which can be helpful in the assessment of the quality of the video. Because of the heterogeneous nature of the content, unstructured and low quality data make KE videos much more challenging. Sports channels use video segmentation techniques to extract useful knowledge from videos. The generation of the subtitle in an automated way is very challenging because of the language barrier and the accent of the individual. This process consists of extraction of audio, speech recognition, decoder, etc. A visual cue can be extracted using facial markers such as the position of the jaw, lips, and nose.

2.4.2 Knowledge Extraction Techniques

As mentioned earlier there are three knowledge extraction techniques, namely the rule-based method (RBM), learning-based method (LBM), and the hybrid method. It is impossible to determine which technique is more efficient and effective in KE. The selection of techniques is totally dependent on the user requirement and the current job. The RBM requires manual rule writing and it is preferred when knowledge is to be presented in a logical way [26,27]. However, it can be static in approach as new rules can be added dynamically as per requirements. The fuzzy approach uses RBM. On the contrary, the LBM is more dynamic. Here, the model is trained based on the available data [28–30]. LBM methods are further categorized into supervised, unsupervised, and semi-supervised learning techniques. The biggest challenge faced by these techniques is handling large and complex datasets. In supervised learning, the training data is labeled. The formation of large-scale data is very time-consuming as well as labor intensive. These techniques can be implemented where specific domain-related knowledge needs to be extracted from the underlying data. The accuracy of these techniques depends on lexical, semantic, morphological, and syntactic factors. In unsupervised learning, labels are not provided. This technique extracts knowledge based on similarity, cluster formation, extraction of knowledge from the text, and relations between entities. In this technique, data preprocessing must be performed with utmost care. If data is dirty or contains noise, then the extracted knowledge can be faulty. In semi-supervised learning, both labeled data and unlabeled data are used with some amount of supervision. Distinct supervised learning, deep learning, and transfer learning techniques are preferred when dealing with larger datasets. Deep-learning techniques show very good results when larger datasets are involved. Deep learning helps in generalization, and unlabeled data is also used. Deep learning possesses an interesting feature that allows it to learn from different hidden layers. Pattern recognition is the best example of the implementation of deep learning. More advanced algorithms can help in achieving higher performance. Self-training can be helpful in eliminating the problem of overfitting. In order to solve large dataset problems, reinforcement learning or supervision with a distant approach can be used. Time series data; unstructured, heterogeneous, and noisy data; and modeling of high dimensional data and its associated performance are some of the challenges that are faced during KE.

REFERENCES

1. Binti Hamzah, F.A., Lau, C., Nazri, H., Ligot, D.V., Lee, G., Tan, C.L. 2020. CoronaTracker: Worldwide COVID-19 Outbreak Data Analysis and Prediction. *Bull World Health Organ. E-pub* 19.
2. McKibbin, W.J., Fernando, R. 2020. The Global Macroeconomic Impacts of COVID-19: Seven Scenarios.
3. Bhattacharjee, Soumyabrata. 2020. Statistical Investigation of the Relationship between the Spread of Coronavirus Disease (COVID-19) and Environmental Factors Based on Study of Four Mostly Affected Places of China and Five Mostly Affected Places of Italy.
4. Teles, P. 2020. Predicting the Evolution of SARS-COVID-2 in Portugal Using an Adapted SIR Model Previously Used in South Korea for the MERS Outbreak. *arXiv Preprint* ArXiv:2003.10047.
5. Liu, P., Beeler, P., Chakrabarty, R.K. 2020. COVID-19 Progression Timeline and Effectiveness of Response-to-Spread Interventions across the United States. *medRxiv.*
6. Li, L., Yang, Z., Dang, Z., Meng, C., Huang, Jet al. 2020. Propagation Analysis and Prediction of the COVID-19. *arXiv Preprint* ArXiv:2003.06846.
7. Lai, S., Bogoch, I.I., Ruktanonchai, N., Watts, A.G., Li, Y., et al. 2020. Assessing Spread Risk of Wuhan Novel Coronavirus within and beyond China, January-April 2020: A Travel Network-Based Modelling Study.
8. Giuliani, D., Dickson, M.M., Espa, G., Santi, F. 2020. Modelling and Predicting the Spread of Coronavirus (COVID-19) Infection in NUTS-3 Italian Regions. *arXiv Preprint* ArXiv:2003.06664.
9. Mahalle, P., Kalamkar, A.B., Dey, N., Chaki, J., Shinde, G.R. 2020. Forecasting Models for Coronavirus (COVID-19): A Survey of the State-of-the-Art.
10. Labrinidis, A., Jagadish, H.V. 2012. Challenges and Opportunities with Big Data. *Proceedings of the VLDB Endowment* 5(12): 2032–2033.

11. Sivarajah, U., Kamal, M.M., Irani, Z., Weerakkody, V. 2017. Critical Analysis of Big Data Challenges and Analytical Methods. *Journal of Business Research* 70: 263–286.
12. Bhadani, A., Jothimani, D. 2016. Big Data: Challenges, Opportunities and Realities. In: Singh, M.K., Kumar, D.G. (Eds.), *Effective Big Data Management and Opportunities for Implementation* (pp. 1–24). Pennsylvania, PA: IGI Global.
13. Nasser, T., Tariq, R.S. 2015. Big Data Challenges. *Journal of Computer Engineering & Information Technology* 4: 3. doi: 10.4172/2324, 9307(2).
14. Jagadish, H.V., Gehrke, J., Labrinidis, A., Papakonstantinou, Y., Patel, J.M., et al. 2014. Big Data and Its Technical Challenges. *Communications of the ACM* 57(7): 86–94.
15. Jaseena, K.U., David, J.M. 2014. Issues, Challenges, and Solutions: Big Data Mining. *CS & IT-CSCP* 4(13): 131–140.
16. Saif, S., Wazir, S. 2018. Performance Analysis of Big Data and Cloud Computing Techniques: A Survey. *Procedia Computer Science* 132: 118–127.
17. Sikeridis, D., Papapanagiotou, I., Rimal, B.P., Devetsikiotis, M. 2017. A Comparative Taxonomy and Survey of Public Cloud Infrastructure Vendors. *arXiv Preprint* ArXiv:1710.01476.
18. Daher, Z., Hajjdiab, H. 2018. Cloud Storage Comparative Analysis Amazon Simple Storage vs. Microsoft Azure Blob Storage. *International Journal of Machine Learning and Computing* 8(1): 85–89.
19. García, S., Ramírez-Gallego, S., Luengo, J., Benítez, J.M., Herrera, F. 2016. Big Data Preprocessing: Methods and Prospects. *Big Data Analytics* 1(1): 9.
20. Zhang, S., Zhang, C., Yang, Q. 2003. Data Preparation for Data Mining. *Applied Artificial Intelligence* 17(5–6): 375–381.
21. Jiang, J. 2012. Information Extraction From Text. In: Aggarwal, C.C. and Zhai, C.X. (Eds.), *Mining Text Data* (pp. 11–41). Boston, MA: Springer.
22. Kim, J.C., Chung, K. 2019. Associative Feature Information Extraction Using Text Mining from Health Big Data. *Wireless Personal Communications* 105(2): 691–707.
23. Zheng, Y., Kong, S., Zhu, W., Ye, H. 2019, December. Scalable Document Image Information Extraction with Application to Domain-Specific Analysis. In: *2019 IEEE International Conference on Big Data (Big Data)* (pp. 5108–5115). IEEE.
24. Manoharan, S. 2019. A Smart Image Processing Algorithm for Text Recognition, Information Extraction and Vocalization for the Visually Challenged. *Journal of Innovative Image Processing (JIIP)* 1(01): 31–38.

25. Skupin, R., Hellge, C., Bross, B., Schierl, T., De La Fuente, Y.S., et al. 2020. U.S. Patent Application No. 16/576,051.
26. Jin, Y., Von Seelen, W., Sendhoff, B. 1998, May. An Approach to Rule-Based Knowledge Extraction. In: *1998 IEEE International Conference on Fuzzy Systems Proceedings (Cat. No. 98CH36228). IEEE World Congress on Computational Intelligence (Cat. No. 98CH36228)* (Vol. 2, pp. 1188–1193). IEEE.
27. Chiticariu, L., Li, Y., Reiss, F. 2013, October. Rule-Based Information Extraction is Dead! Long Live Rule-Based Information Extraction Systems! In: *Proceedings of the 2013 Conference on Empirical Methods in Natural Language Processing* (pp. 827–832).
28. Adnan, K., Akbar, R. 2019. An Analytical Study of Information Extraction from Unstructured and Multidimensional Big Data. *Journal of Big Data* 6(1), 91.
29. Holzinger, A., Kieseberg, P., Tjoa, A.M., Weippl, E. 2017. *Machine Learning and Knowledge Extraction*. Hamburg, Germany: Springer.
30. Bao, X., Xie, S., Zhang, K., Song, K., Yang, Y. 2019, November. Machine Learning Based Information Extraction for Diabetic Nephropathy in Clinical Text Documents. In: *2019 6th International Conference on Systems and Informatics (ICSAI)* (pp. 1438–1442). IEEE.

BIG DATA ANALYTICS
FOR COVID-19

3.1 ALL YOU NEED TO KNOW

This section briefs the basic skills and terminologies required for data analytics. Apart from technical skills, analytical skills like critical thinking and problem-solving are also required for a successful data scientist.

3.1.1 WEB 2.0

In this digital era, weather forecasting, stock market analysis, and e-shopping are very easy as these are visualized in such a way that a layman can easily annotate with an interactive digital platform. This progress took years to shape before the user could retrieve information from the World Wide Web (WWW); however, information was in static form using only text and multimedia. This information can be accessed through Google network and it was referred to the web through which information can be fetched. Using the web, users can listen to audio, can watch animations, and can even see virtual environments. Users can also transfer a file from one computer to another using the web [1]. Analysts and researchers found the need for online interactive participation in view of content creation and visualization. With this need, Web 2.0 emerged as an interactive/social web platform where people can communicate online with each other. Web 2.0 provides the facility of semantic tagging which results in effective searching and recommendations [2,3]. There is always the need for the human aspect alongside textual information, which is fulfilled by Web 2.0. Various technologies and platforms are provided by Web 2.0 that are helpful for social networking. few of the most popular platforms are as follows:

- **Blogs:** This is the online platform for sharing of information where others can interact with the host of the data through comments.

- **Wikis:** This provides a platform to seamlessly edit, share, and add information on web pages.
- **Flickr:** This provides the facility of tagging any image with information; it is useful for sharing photos.
- **Google Docs:** Using Google Docs, word documents can be easily shared with a group of people for inline updating.
- **Twitter:** This is an interactive blogging platform where people can share their thoughts and others can also put in their views.

3.1.2 Critical Thinking

Various data storage platforms are provided by service providers to store big data and to provide services for data analytics as presented in Chapter 2 of this book. There is a need to have analytical and critical thinking to extract knowledge from such big data. Critical thinking can improve the quality of predictions, and accurate predictions can increase the revenue of that organization and other benefits of the business. Accurate predictions of pandemic diseases like COVID-19 can save human lives globally, which is invaluable. Hence, critical thinking plays an important role in data analytics, and this is one of the skills every data scientist should possess [4]. Critical thinking involves:

- The ability to recognize the complications of effective analysis
- The ability to understand the restrictions of analysis
- The ability to deliberate uncertainty

A data scientist needs to understand the requirements and benefits of data analysis, and this can be done by preparing a questionnaire [5]. A sample set of questions is listed below:

- How unique will the result provided by this analysis be?
- How are other researchers looking at this data analysis?
- Is there any parameter that I am missing?
- Are there any other conclusions other than this analysis?
- When to stop analyzing? When to conclude?
- Do I provide correct explanations?
- Am I exaggerating conclusions?
- What are the benefits of the analysis?
- Who will benefit from this analysis?
- What are the data sources?

This questionnaire can help to understand analysis with unique results and also be useful to the broad range of audiences.

3.1.3 Statistical Programming (R/Python)

In data science, statistics plays a dominant role as it uses mathematics for analyzing data. Various visualization tools can be used to view data in different aspects; however, to understand data and to take out the meaning from data mathematics is necessary [6]. The conclusions of the data analysis are more concrete and trustworthy when the analysis is done using mathematics. Data analysis results need to be accurate to increase revenue, and in a situation like COVID-19 it can save precious human life. Mathematical analysis of data can provide a deeper understanding and insight into the data. Modern data analysis algorithms, i.e. ML algorithms, are based on mathematics and statistics; hence, to understand the theory behind these algorithms, knowledge of statistics is important. Statistics is used to solve multifaceted real-world problems using mathematics. Hence, in data analytics there is a need for programming languages that can support statistics. There are various languages and tools that support statistical operations, e.g. R, SAS, Python, Julia, and SPSS, and among these R and Python are used widely around the globe due to their numerous benefits [7].

3.1.4 R Programming Language

R is a statistical programming language used for data analytics, and it provides the facility of easy integration with languages like C++, SQL, and Java [8]. It was initially developed keeping in mind academicians and researchers as target customers; however, due to its features it is also well received by companies in software development. The features and benefits of R are as follows:

- It is a free programming language which provides a statistical environment.
- It provides almost all ML algorithms, e.g. clustering, classification, and regression.
- It supports numerical calculations for plotting charts.
- It can be used in almost all platforms, e.g. Windows, Unix, FreeBSD, MacOS, and Linux.
- It can easily be integrated with languages like C, C++, Java, and SQL.

- It is an interpreted language and provides better community support.
- It is very simple to learn and use.

R provides various features and benefits for academicians, researchers, and industries; however, this has memory management and security issues. It does not support a pure object-oriented programming nature as Python.

3.1.5 Python Programming Language

Python is a general-purpose language as it can be used for data analytics, game development, implementing websites, and as an OOP programming language. It provides vast numbers of functionalities for performing ML algorithms, websites, and game development, e.g. libraries like Pandas, Numpy, Scipy, and TensorFlow and platforms like Flask and Django to name a few [9]. The features of Python are as follows:

- It is an open source and free language.
- It provides various functionalities to collect, process, analyze, and view data of various formats.
- It provides Graphical User Interface (GUI); hence, it is easy to handle.
- It is an interpreted and portable language.
- It supports OOP; hence, it can easily integrate with OOP languages like C++ and Java.
- It can be used for game and web development applications.
- It has the huge support of libraries.

Python grabbed the market rapidly due to its ease of use and support of various libraries. Scientists can easily analyze their research using Python without requiring detailed knowledge about programming using the abstraction feature.

3.2 DATA VISUALIZATION

Data visualization is as important as data analysis. Organizations invest much time and money for data analysis as data is in high volume, and analyzing voluminous data requires the use of various complex algorithms. Retrieving, cleaning, and preparing data are the prerequisites of data analysis, and these phases need ample amounts of valuable time. Results are obtained after completing the data processing phases, and if these results are in a format that is too complex to understand, then the organization may not get the benefits out of the huge investment. Textual information always takes much time to understand than graphical information, as graphical content grabs the attention of the human brain more than textual information. Data visualization doesn't mean just displaying information using graphs and charts; it is providing correct information with appropriate visualization methods. There are various visualization tools used in data analytics, i.e. Tableau, Qlik Sense, and Power BI [10].

3.2.1 Big Data Analytics and COVID-19

3.2.1.1 Statistical Parameters

The quality of data analysis and the accuracy of prediction are majorly dependent on the parameters selected for data analysis. In the case of the recent COVID-19 pandemic, predictions can help to minimize the spread rate and death rate. In the initial period of COVID-19, predictions were estimated based on the duration and count of infection/death. The COVID-19 infection spread globally, and the number of infections increased in huge numbers; researchers tried to search various parameters that can impact the infection rate. Mobility is a major factor in increasing the infection rate; when people come in the vicinity of an infected person, then through his/her droplets, infection can increase [11,12]. Social distancing can control the infection rate; hence, in many countries/cities people follow social distancing [13,14]. Researchers are also trying to find the impact of metrological parameters, e.g. temperature, humidity, and wind speed on the infection rate [15–18]. Patients' ages, genders, and medical histories also have an impact on COVID-19 infection [19,20]. Similarly, these parameters can be categorized into four types: social, metrological, disease-related, and patient-related. The parameters and this classification are depicted in Figure 3.1:

3.2.1.2 Predictive Analytics

Forecasting of COVID-19 infection/death count is required as it is growing in a faster range. Predictive analysis can be used to forecast

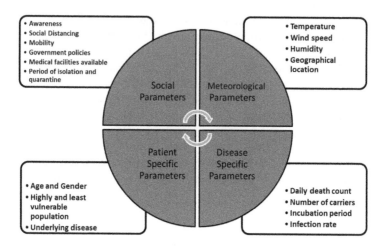

Figure 3.1 Categories of COVID-19 parameters.

the infection count and accordingly precautions can be taken by people, healthcare workers, and the government. As discussed in the above section, various parameters can impact the infection rate; hence, there must be prediction methods that can take these parameters as the base of the analysis. Broadly, there are two major categories of prediction methods [21]:

- Mathematical and Stochastic Theory
- Learning Models

In the mathematical/stochastic theory, the Susceptible-Infection-Recovered (SIR) model is used for predictions. In the literature, extended SIR models are also presented [22,23]. Using these models, predictions can be done. However, mathematical models are not useful for data that changes with time. In such a case, COVID-19 data is changing faster; here learning models will be well suited for predictions [24,25]. However, there are various learning models, and among these, selection of the appropriate model can impact on the quality of the predictions.

3.3 DATA MODELS AND PERFORMANCE

Building data models and performance assessment play a crucial role in data analytics. This section discusses data modeling in detail along with the assessment of data model performance.

3.3.1 Data Modeling Phases

The application of data analytics techniques on big data is a repetitive process. Uncovering patterns, establishing correlations, applying statistics, building models, and testing and deployment are the main steps in data analytics. Data modeling is a core activity in the process of data analytics. It repetitively applies any ML technique to identify the model which best fits the business. Selecting the best performing model is the crucial step in data analytics, and data modeling can be effectively done using R programming or SaS. Visualization and communication are also important steps in data modeling which include tools like Tableau, Power BI, and QlickView for better presentation, as discussed earlier. Key steps in building data science models are described below [26]:

i. **Setting Goals**

Setting up the goals and the questions to be addressed after model deployment is the first and most crucial step in building a data model. It should be noted that this is an uncertain and hypothetical step in the initial phase and is to be executed with the utmost care. Deciding the scope, risk factors, mitigation strategies, and business targets are also part of this step.

ii. **Communication**

Users, data scientists, support team, legal compliance, and business drivers are the main stakeholders in building data models. It is very important to initiate communication between all the stakeholders for common agreement on the functional and execution issues. All these stakeholders play an equally important role in the deployment phase to fix up the bugs, if any. Change management, regular updates, and alignment, if any, are also part of this step.

iii. **Exploratory Data Analysis**

Most of the time, the dataset received consists of missing values and is messy. It is very important to decide which values should replace these missing values or inconsistent entries. In this step, the dataset is analyzed as an initial investigation to consolidate the main features of the dataset with the help of visualization. Anomalies detection, hypothesis testing, and pattern discovery are also carried out in this step.

iv. **Functional Forming**

Deciding the nature of the dataset, whether it is continuous, discrete, or binary, fixing the dependent variable, i.e. the target variable, its nature (binary or in another form), and the distribution of this dependent variable are the major functionalities of this phase.

v. **Data Splitting**

Prediction is an important outcome of any data analytic technique. However, how we divide this data into training and testing sets also decides the performance of the underlying model. The training dataset is used to build the model and the testing dataset is used to validate the model. This dataset splitting plays a very important role in model validation. The stability of the model is an important feature, which means that the model should behave approximately the same over time.

vi. **Model Performance**

As mentioned earlier, stability is the most important metric for the assessment of model performance. Another metric is the accuracy of predictions generated by the model and its comparison with the real values. Fitting of the model, the significance of the predicted values or predictions, the correlation between the dependent variable and the predictor, as well as their comparison with the benchmarked model are also part of model assessment.

vii. **Model Deployment**

Deploying the final model and its testing with different test cases are important steps in this phase. Representational State Transfer (REST) Application Programming Interfaces (APIs) can be used to send data in JSON format, which is an encoded format, to test against the model to decide whether any change management is required for the next step.

viii. **Model Re-building**

Re-building of the model is required in many unexpected circumstances, which include underperformance of the model, inaccurate predictions, change in the platform, and loss of variables used for forming the functions.

Major roles in data modeling are depicted in Figure 3.2.

3.3.2 Ensemble Data Model

When an individual data model does not provide accurate predictions or underperforms, then the ensemble data model is used to improve the performance. In the ensemble data model, different models are

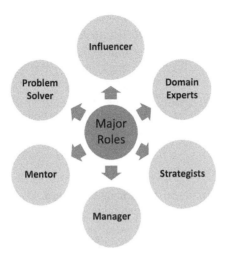

Figure 3.2 Major roles in data modeling.

trained and created and then combined together to improve the results. In the ensemble data model, sometimes multiple modeling algorithms are used or different training datasets are used for improvement in the outcome. An appropriate aggregation method is then used to combine the outcome of the individual model, either by the method of averaging or majority voting. Optimizing generalization in the prediction due to noise, bias, and variance and improving the stability of the model is the main motivation behind the ensemble model. The reason is that the base models used in the ensemble techniques are not dependent and are varied [26].

Consider the scenario where you have developed a mobile application for creating awareness about COVID-19 and improving the immune system to alleviate the infection of COVID-19. Before launching this mobile application for use in society, it would be good to request suggestions and feedback in order to improve and fine-tune this application further. In this case, we can divide our contacts into a few clusters in order to take feedback or release a beta version. These clusters are listed as follows:

1. Family and close friends
2. Professional contacts
3. Contact from social networks
4. Release of the beta version

Naturally, the release of the beta version will be a more effective idea to receive correct and live feedback about your application. However, combining critical suggestions from all the four categories listed above will surely improve the pool of suggestions in all respects. These suggestions received from multiple users and multi-aged groups will help further in fine-tuning and fixing the bugs in your mobile application before the final release. As discussed, the same concept is used in the ensemble data model to improve the results and predictions.

3.3.3 Model Performance

As stated earlier, model performance is based on various parameters. Further, the following techniques can also be used for model improvement [26].

a. **Meta-modeling**

In meta-modeling, the outcome from multiple sub-models is combined in a specific order to present the meta-model of the entire ecosystem.

b. **Boosting**

In boosting, weights of values under consideration are varied iteratively based on the previous classification. This process is carried out vice versa if the accuracy of classification is not as expected. This technique is used for better predictive accuracy.

c. **Bagging**

Bagging uses an ensemble model where each model is given a different subset of the dataset as input and finally the combined output is considered as an output of the overall model. Random forest algorithm uses the method of boosting to improve performance.

3.4 BIG DATA TECHNIQUES

With an increasing number of devices connected to the Internet witnessing the notion of the Internet of Things (IoT) [27,28] and the sudden onset of the COVID-19 pandemic [21] in early 2020 is contributing massively to the big data. This big data is mainly driven by smart devices, IoT, AI, and social networks. Some of the prominent challenges in analyzing this big data are a combination of old and new technologies, backward and upward interoperability with the tools and technologies, scale, and pace. In addition to this, an environment where there is a lack of standards in data interoperability, security and privacy are other important challenges. In a nutshell, when data becomes big, the legacy methods of data analytics do not work efficiently. The main aim of this section is to discuss the techniques to explore and analyze this big data, how to process the data, as well as get meaningful insights from this data. The main big data analytics techniques are described below.

3.4.1 Association Rule Learning

Example: Underlying secondary diseases in patients with COVID-19 may lead to mortality.

Discussion: Considering the example stated above, the association rule learning technique is used when the dataset consists of logical interrelations between multiple columns or features. This technique is useful to explore the correlation among various columns of a database or dataset. This technique uses a rule-based (if/then or if/then/else) mechanism to infer the associations or logical connections between various columns or features in the dataset. Support and confidence are the two main patterns majorly used by this technique in order to find semantic similarities. Apriori, Eclat, and F-P growth algorithms [29] are popular algorithms used for association rule learning.

3.4.2 Classification Tree Analysis

Example: The disease under discussion belongs to which category?

Discussion: This technique is widely used in computing data analytics and mining and in statistical modeling. When we work on a huge dataset consisting of the details of underlined application and new observation or reading comes in, this technique is used to decide the category of this new observation. This technique requires trained (i.e. accurately collected observations) past data for classification. This technique is applicable to both structured as well as unstructured datasets. Classification can be binary classification, multi-class classification, or multi-label classification, and it is carried as per the underlined application. Initializing the required classifier, training it, predicting the target feature, and then evaluating this classifier for the required performance metrics are major steps in using the classification model. K-nearest neighbor and decision trees are some examples of classification techniques [30].

3.4.3 Genetic Algorithm

Example: Which medicine should we recommend to COVID-19 patients and at which stage to optimize the recovery period?

Discussion: Genetics algorithms are mainly applied to an optimization problem where the objective is to either maximize or minimize some criterion function. As stated in the example, this approach can be efficiently applied to optimize the recovery period of COVID-19-infected patients by recommending proper medicines. Inheritance, mutation, and selection are the three main steps in using a genetics algorithm to solve the optimization problem. This approach can also be used for feature selection with the help of methods like filter method, wrapper method, or embedded method. The main advantage of a genetics algorithm is that it performs better for a large feature set, and it is computationally efficient as compared to other approaches. Resource allocation, investment decision-making, cargo loading problems, etc., are some examples of problems that can be efficiently solved using genetic algorithms [31].

3.4.4 Machine Learning

Example: Which hospital from the authorized list would the patient prefer next time, based on their experience?

Discussion: Machine Learning (ML) includes two components, i.e. a machine and learning. The machine is a computing device with memory, battery, and computational power. Learning is obtaining and refining performance from past experience. ML is a process of programming computers for optimizing outcomes using a dataset of underlying applications or historical data or experience. The main objective of ML is to design and develop new optimization algorithms and techniques that will enable computers to learn from use cases or past data. It is equally important to understand when we require ML techniques. The following are some ideal situations where we need ML.

i.   When it is challenging and computationally inefficient to program the computers to perform the task.
ii. Where human skills and expertise cannot be made available.
iii. Where humans are helpless to express their knowledge and capabilities.

iv. Problems where the solutions are dynamic.
v. When the data is big and traditional approaches are not adequate.

ML is used when the outcome of the problem is prediction, learning, decision making, remembering, recognition, or analysis [26].

3.4.5 Regression Analysis

Example: How does the income of the patient affect the class of hospital he/she prefers?

Discussion: Regression analysis is the method of finding the line for fitting the best for a given dataset of target use cases. It is the process of manipulating the value of some independent variable which can represent, for example, the income of the patient, to observe how it changes the preference of selecting the class of hospital. This technique explains how the value of the dependent variable varies with respect to the change in the value of the independent variable and is more appropriate for the datasets consisting of continuous values. For example, in linear regression, the error is calculated as shown in Equation 3.1.

$$\text{Error} = \text{Actual Value} - \text{Predicted Value} \qquad (3.1)$$

This method calculates residuals which are the difference between the actual and estimated values of the function calculated based on the training data. Mathematically, the residual is presented in Equation 3.2.

$$\varepsilon_i = f(x_i) - \hat{f}(x_i) \qquad (3.2)$$

3.4.6 Social Network Analysis

Example: How many degrees of connect does a patient have to find blood donors?

Discussion: As the number of users on online social networks like Facebook and Twitter is increasing at a faster rate, the social network analysis techniques are becoming more popular for big data analytics. There are many use cases like recommender system, understanding social connect of customers, the relationship amongst the customer base where the use of social network analysis is more effective by adopting the concept of community behavior. The graph data structure is the most potential data structure used in this technique where the vertex represents an entity or individual in the network, and an edge connecting the vertex represents the connection or relationship between these entities. The main measure of social network analysis is centrality that calculates the most powerful or significant person in the graph and is calculated using the in-degree and out-degree. It is generally represented by a score.

3.5 BIG DATA TOOLS AND TECHNOLOGY

There are various open source tools for data analysis. Data analysis is done on big data which practically needs various services like data storage, data warehouse, and tools for data extraction, data cleaning, and data visualization [32]. The traditional data management strategies are not enough to handle such high volume and heterogeneous data; hence, there is a need for tools that can support big data processing functionalities. The big data tools are listed in Table 3.1. Many of these are open source and free tools. Open source tools are widely used by the big data community due to the huge online support available.

- **Data Collection Tools:** Data collection is the first step in data analytics. The Semantria tool provides facilities to collect data from various clients with text analytics. This is a customizable tool that is easy for operating. Opinion Crawl and Open Text provide the facility of sentiment analysis on the data of websites. Trackur also works on sentiment analysis to collect data from online social media networks. SAS uses sentiment analysis on real-time data and provides automated charts based on patterns in the real-time data.
- **Data Storage Tools:** Apache provides various storage tools for structured and unstructured data, i.e. Apache HBase, Apache Cassandra, Apache Ignite, and CouchDB. In many applications data doesn't follow any schema; for such data MongoDB storage is used. It is lightweight and is based on JSON.
- **Data Extraction and Filtering Tools:** These are web scrapping tools. These tools provide facilities to capture unstructured information from the internet and convert it into a structured

TABLE 3.1
Summary of Big Data Tools

			Big Data Tools			
Sr. No	Data Collection	Data Storage	Data Extraction and Filtering	Data Cleaning	Data Analytics	Data Visualization
1	Semantria	Apache HBase	Spinn3r	DataCleaner	Hive	Tbleau
2	Opinion Crawl	CouchDB	OctoParse	MapRecuce	Apache Spark	Qlik
3	OpenText	MongoDB	Webhose.io	Rapidminer	Apache Storm	Orange
4	Trackur	Apache Cassandra	Mozenda	OpenRefine	Qubole	Google Fusion tables
5	SAS Sentiment Analysis	Apache Ignite	Content Grabber	Talend	Flink	CartoDB

format, i.e. Mozenda and Octoparse. Webhose.io provides the facility of extracting data for a particular duration from online sites and converts it into a structured format. Spinn3r can be used to extract data from online social media networks and keeps data in the form of JSON files. Content Grabber can be used to extract data from multiple sources and can be saved in Excel, CSV, or XML formats.

- **Data Cleaning Tools:** Rapidminer, OpenRefine, and Talend are data cleaning tools. These help to minimize the time required for data processing. DataCleaner is integrated with Hadoop and provides various data cleaning operations, e.g. finding duplicate values, transformations, and pattern discovery. Apache provides various data analytics tools such as Hive, Apache Spark, Apache Storm, and Flink.

- **Data Analytics Tools:** Big data analytics tools provide various capabilities of data analysis like predictive analysis, neural networks, etc. In many applications there may be a requirement of using more than one tool and, hence, integration with other tools is the most important feature of big data analytics tools. As data may change dynamically in every aspect, like size and format, these tools should be scalable and should be able to adapt such heterogeneous high-volume data. In some applications analysis may be done on an organization's sensitive data; hence, the security of data is important. Data analytics tools should provide secure data access as data is big in volume. Hence, for faster analysis these tools should provide batch or stream analytics for parallel execution. There are various data analytics tools provided by Apache, e.g. Hive, Spark, Storm, and Flink.

- **Data Visualization Tools:** Data visualization is important as much as data analytics, and the result must be in a format that can be easily understood. Visualization tools like Tableau, Qlik, Orange, Google Fusion tables, and CartoDB provide the facility of providing analytics results in graphical formats. As discussed earlier, graphical representation makes it very easy to understand the complex results. A summary of these big data tools is presented in Table 3.1.

To build any data analytics application, we require data analytics technologies. Data analytics technologies can be divided into two categories, i.e. operational big data and analytical big data. Operational data technologies process the data that is generated by day-to-day operations, e.g. online shopping, ticket bookings, social media like Facebook, Twitter, etc. Analytical big data technologies work on complex data instead of operational data, and based on this analysis essential real-time business decisions can be taken. Further, these technologies can be categorized based on the big data functionality provided by them, i.e. data storage, data mining, data analytics, and data visualization. Various data analytics technologies are emerging such as Blockchain, TensorFlow, Beam and Airflow, Apache Kafka, Kubernetes, and Docker [32,33].

- **Blockchain:** This is used for secure payments and provides privacy of data, and financial frauds can be minimized as it possesses a secure architecture and also provides faster transactions. It is used globally for financial transactions. Real-time data analysis can be done using Blockchains. Banks can keep an eye on changes in real-time data and abnormal transactions with Blockchains, and can make quick decisions. Data scientists can use the computational power of multiple computers that are connected through the Blockchain network for extensive forecasting. Data used for analysis may not be used repeatedly for predictions on which data analysis already is done and predictions are made by some other scientists. Hence, predictions of one team can be useful to others and they can make progress instead of doing the same task again. However, data storage on the blockchain is expensive than other storage solutions. The Blockchain technology was developed by bitcoin using C++, Python, and JavaScript languages. It is used by a number of organizations, e.g. Facebook, Metlife, and Oracle.
- **TensorFlow:** This was developed by Google Brain Team in Python and C++ languages using CUDA. It is a library that is used to develop and deploy ML applications. It provides simple and readable syntax; hence, application development and deployment are not a complex task. The execution model of TensorFlow provides the facility of implementing and executing a single graph. Due to this modularization, many applications can be built efficiently. TensorBoard provides visualization of the application execution on the web-based dashboard. TensorFlow provides a better facility of debugging; here the developer can debug single graphs separately and then debug the entire graph. It has extensive ML community support. Due

to these advantages, it is used globally by various organizations, e.g. Intel, eBay, Airbnb, and Google.

* **Apache Beam:** Apache Beam was developed for building and managing a parallel data processing pipeline for faster execution. It provides both batch and stream data processing. Big data can be chopped in chunks and can be processed in parallel. The biggest advantage of using a beam is that developers can use any SDK (Python or Java) for programming logic; hence, it is comfortable for developing any data analytics application. It is developed in Python and JAVA language. It is used by organizations such as Amazon, Oracle, and Cisco.

* **Kafka:** Apache provides real-time data streaming tools for data analytics, i.e. Kafka. Kafka works as a distributed streaming platform like a message queue. Clusters of Kafka store records in publisher streams and these are categorized according to topics. Publisher APIs are provided for applications to publish their data according to the topics of Kafka, and to access these records, consumer APIs are provided. Records can be searched easily based on the "topic" and, hence, data access is faster. Kafka provides higher throughput and low latency and is a scalable platform for data analytics. Due to these facilities, Kafka is used by various organizations like Netflix, Twitter, and Yahoo.

REFERENCES

1. O'Reilly, T. 2007. What Is Web 2.0: Design patterns and business models for the next generation of software. *Communications & Strategies* 17(1): 1–5. https://www.oreilly.com/pub/a/web2/archive/what-is-web-20.html.
2. Murugesan, S. 2007. Understanding Web 2.0. *IT Professional* 9(4): 34–41. doi: 10.1109/MITP.2007.78.
3. Cormode, G., Krishnamurthy, B. 2008. Key Differences Between Web 1.0 and Web 2.0. *First Monday* 13(6).
4. McKinney, E., Niese, B. 2016. *Big Data Critical Thinking Skills for Analysts - Learning to Ask the Right Questions.* AMCIS.
5. Rasheva-Yordanova, K., Iliev, E., Nikolova, B. 2018, July. Analytical Thinking as A Key Competence for Overcoming the Data Science Divide. In: *Proceedings of the EDULEARN18 Conference* (pp. 2–4).
6. Louridas, P., Ebert, C. 2013. Embedded Analytics and Statistics for Big Data. *IEEE Software* 30(6): 33–39.
7. Siddiqui, T., Alkadri, M., Khan, N.A. 2017. Review of Programming Languages and Tools for Big Data Analytics. *International Journal of Advanced Research & Computer Science* 8(5): 1112–1118.

8. Farhad Malik, R. Statistical Programming Language. https://to
   wardsdatascience.com/r-statistical-programming-language-6adc
   8c0a6e3d [Accessed: 20-April-2020].
9. Ozgur, C., Colliau, T., Rogers, G., Hughes, Z., Myer-Tyson, B.
   2017. MATLAB vs. Python vs. R. *Journal of Data Science* 15(3):
   355–372.
10. Caldarola, E.G., Rinaldi, A.M. 2017, July. Big Data Visualization
    Tools: A Survey. In: *Proceedings of the 6th International Conference
    on Data Science, Technology and Applications* (pp. 296–305).
    SCITEPRESS-Science and Technology Publications, Lda.
11. Siegenfeld, A.F., Bar-Yam, Y. 2020. Eliminating COVID-19: A
    Community-Based Analysis. *arXiv Preprint* ArXiv:2003.10086.
12. Liu, P., Beeler, P., Chakrabarty, R.K. 2020. COVID-19 Progression
    Timeline and Effectiveness of Response-to-Spread Interventions
    across the United States. *medRxiv.*
13. Bayham, J., Fenichel, E.P. 2020. The Impact of School Closure for
    COVID-19 on the US Healthcare Workforce and the Net Mortality
    Effects. *medRxiv.*
14. Sameni, R. 2020. Mathematical Modeling of Epidemic Diseases:
    A Case Study of the COVID-19 Coronavirus. *arXiv preprint
    arXiv:2003.11371.*
15. Bhattacharjee, S. 2020. Statistical Investigation of Relationship
    between Spread of Coronavirus Disease (COVID-19) and
    Environmental Factors Based on Study of Four Mostly Affected
    Places of China and Five Mostly Affected Places of Italy. *arXiv
    preprint arXiv:2003.11277.*
16. Chen, B., Liang, H., Yuan, X., Hu, Y., Xu, M., et al. 2020. Roles
    of Meteorological Conditions in COVID-19 Transmission on a
    Worldwide Scale. *medRxiv.*
17. Ma, Y., Zhao, Y., Liu, J., He, X., Wang, B., et al. 2020. Effects of
    Temperature Variation and Humidity on the Mortality of COVID-
    19 in Wuhan. *medRxiv.*
18. Shi, P., Dong, Y., Yan, H., Li, X., Zhao, C., et al. 2020. The Impact
    of Temperature and Absolute Humidity on the Coronavirus disease
    2019 (COVID-19) Outbreak-Evidence from China. *medRxiv.*
19. Dowd, J.B., Rotondi, V., Adriano, L., Brazel, D.M., Block, P., et al.
    2020. Demographic Science Aids in Understanding the Spread and
    Fatality Rates of COVID-19. *medRxiv.*
20. DeCaprio, D., Gartner, J., Burgess, T., Kothari, S., Sayed, S.
    2020. Building a COVID-19 Vulnerability Index. *arXiv Preprint*
    ArXiv:2003.07347.
21. Shinde, Gitanjali R., Kalamkar, Asmita B., Mahalle, Parikshit
    N., Dey, Nilanjan, Chaki, Jyotismita, Hassanien, Aboul ella
    2020. Forecasting Models for Coronavirus (COVID-19): A
    Survey of the State-of-the-Art. *TechRxiv.* Preprint. doi:10.36227/
    techrxiv.12101547.v1.

22. Teles, P. 2020. Predicting the Evolution of SARS-Covid-2 in Portugal Using an Adapted SIR Model Previously Used in South Korea for the MERS Outbreak. *arXiv Preprint* ArXiv:2003.10047.
23. Victor, A. 2020. Mathematical Predictions for COVID-19 as a Global Pandemic. Available at SSRN 3555879.
24. Mahalle, Parikshit, N., Sable, Nilesh, P., Mahalle, Namita, P., Shinde, Gitanjali, R. 2020. Predictive Analytics of COVID-19 Using Information, Communication and Technologies. Preprints 2020, 2020040257. doi:10.20944/preprints202004.0257.v1.
25. Fong, S.J., Li, G., Dey, N., Crespo, R.G., Herrera-Viedma, E. 2020. Finding an Accurate Early Forecasting Model from Small Dataset: A Case of 2019-Ncov Novel Coronavirus Outbreak. *arXiv Preprint* ArXiv:2003.10776.
26. Bishop, Christopher M. 2006. *Pattern Recognition and Machine Learning* (pp. 315, 520). New York, NY: Springer-Verlag.
27. Mahalle, Parikshit N. 2013. Identity Management Framework for Internet of Things PhD dissertation. Denmark: Aalborg University.
28. Shinde, Gitanjali, Olesen, Henning 2015, April. Interaction Between Users and IoT Clusters: Moving Towards an internet of People, Things and Services (IoPTS). In: *WWRF 34th Meeting, 21st -23rd April 2015*, Santa Clara, CA.
29. Gashaw, Y., Fang, L. 2018. Performance Evaluation of Frequent Pattern Mining Algorithms Using Web Log Data for Web Usage Mining. In: *International Congress on Image & Signal Processing*.
30. Chandre, P.R., Mahalle, P.N., Shinde, G.R. 2018, November. Machine Learning Based Novel Approach for Intrusion Detection and Prevention System: A Tool Based Verification. In: *2018 IEEE Global Conference on Wireless Computing and Networking (GCWCN)* (pp. 135–140). IEEE.
31. Ezugwu, A.E., Pillay, V., Hirasen, D., Sivanarain, K., Govender, M. 2019. A Comparative Study of Meta-Heuristic Optimization Algorithms for 0 – 1 Knapsack Problem: Some Initial Results. *IEEE Access* 7: 43979–44001.
32. Ramadan, R.A. 2017. Big Data Tools-an Overview. *International Journal of Computer & Software Engineering* 2017: 125.
33. Paik, Hye-Young, Xu, Xiwei, Bandara, Dilum, Lee, Sung, Lo, Sin Kuang. 2019. Analysis of Data Management in Blockchain-Based Systems: From Architecture to Governance. *IEEE Access*: 1–1. doi:10.1109/ACCESS.2019.2961404.

MITIGATION STRATEGIES AND RECOMMENDATIONS

4.1 CASE STUDIES OF COVID-19 OUTBREAK: GLOBAL SCENARIO

An outbreak of the novel COVID-19 disease was first observed in Wuhan, China. Soon after that this virus spread across the globe. Efforts toward containment of the disease are being exercised. Countries are locking down their borders until further notice. Lockdowns have restricted movement of people, which has helped in the containment of the virus. In this chapter we are going to study the global scenario related to COVID-19. In addition to it, mitigation strategies and recommendations for the general public and patients are discussed.

The case studies selected for the global scenarios include countries which are majorly affected by the disease.

The selected case studies for this purpose are as follows:

(i) COVID-19 spread in China
(ii) COVID-19 spread in Italy
(iii) COVID-19 spread in the United States

4.1.1 COVID-19 Spread in China

We will start with the first case study, i.e. COVID-19 spread in China. COVID-19 just took 30 days to spread from Wuhan, Hubei province, to Mainland China. After analyzing the initial cases of the outbreak, it was clear that the virus was highly contagious. Extreme measures were taken by the Chinese government to contain the spread of the virus. The measures included complete shutdown, isolation, lockdown of cities, enforcing work from homemeasures, shutdown of schools and colleges, massive construction of hospitals, etc. Even after all this, the virus took over large areas in very little time.

A majority of the infected patients were males aged 30–69. Of these, which is 51.4%, 22% were farmers and laborers. Most of the cases reported were the result of Wuhan-related exposure (85.8%). These were the registered cases at the initial stage of the pandemic. As of April 22, 2020, according to WHO, the total number of confirmed cases in China was 84,287 of which 4,642 was the death count [1].

4.1.2 COVID-19 Spread in Italy

Italy witnessed the beginning of the epidemic by the end of January 2020 when a few Chinese tourists in Rome were found to be COVID-19 positive. The outbreak was first observed in Lombardy. After that the virus progressed slowly, covering a wide geographical area with each passing day. As the condition began to worsen, more critical extraordinary measures were taken by the government to stop the spread. Complete lockdown and shutdown of all industrial and commercial areas were implemented. The average age of deceased patients was 81. Most of the patients were having one or more underlying diseases. As of April 22, 2020, according to WHO, the total number of confirmed cases in Italy was 183,957 of which 24,648 was the death count [2–4].

4.1.3 COVID-19 Spread in the United States

As previously mentioned, the virus is highly contagious. The number of people infected in the United States escalated very quickly. As of April 22, 2020, according to WHO, the total number of confirmed cases in the United States was 776,907, of which 37,602 was the death count. The age group between 65 and 85 was at the highest risk of experiencing the severe symptoms of COVID-19. Patients who were experiencing the symptoms were also having one or more underlying disease conditions. The most commonly reported conditions were diabetes mellitus, chronic lung disease, and cardiovascular disease. These findings are congruent with that of China and Italy [5–7].

4.2 MITIGATION STRATEGIES AND DISCUSSION

This outbreak has impacted the world economy in the worst possible way. As countries that are majorly affected are on lockdowns, the production rate in these countries has been decreased. This has

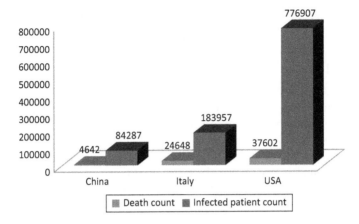

Figure 4.1 Statistics of infected patients and the death count.

affected the GDPs of the nations. This pandemic is going to change the definition of "normal."

From the global scenario it is visible that this virus is spreading across the world at an unprecedented rate. After the initial outbreak, either community transmission or cluster transmission was observed. Figure 4.1 gives the statistics of these three countries. The rate of COVID-19 infection and death count is increasing at a faster rate.

In order to stop the virus spread, community mitigation should be applied. Community mitigation refers to the steps taken by the people or communities to stop the spread of the virus. Community mitigation is very important before a vaccine is developed. The main aim behind community mitigation is to stop the spread of the virus and to protect the people who are at higher risk of getting infected. The protection of healthcare professionals is also very important.

As each community has different population demographics, and the work culture associated with it, community mitigation strategies can vary. These strategies can be implemented according to the situation faced by that particular community. Before implementation of the strategies, it is very important for communities to identify all the necessary services and consider how to implement them efficiently and effectively during this period. Lack of necessary services can cause havoc among the public [8].

It is important that people should know the severity of the situation so that the guidelines set by the authorities will be followed by the communities. Strict action can be taken against persons who do not follow these guidelines.

4.3 ISSUES AND CHALLENGES

The COVID-19 situation quickly escalated into a pandemic in much less time than expected. In this situation, an aid from forecasting models will be very handy. These models can help in essentially getting the forecast of the situation. If the situation is known, then the preparation for the forthcoming situation can be done. But these forecasting models face various challenges. One of the biggest challenges faced by these models is the unavailability of data in a proper format. If data is accurate, so will be the prediction. But if not, it can lead to results which are not true. The next logical step is to convert the data into a proper format. It means to clean the data and essentially deal with missing entries. Cleaning data is an essential and crucial step, but too clean data sometimes loses its integrity, which can lead to a problematic situation. The next step is to select an algorithm for the forecasting. If the algorithm selected is correct, it can give accurate results; if the selection is wrong, the results can be devastating. Also, the model selected should not be too simple or too complex. Overfitting of the data is also one of the biggest concerns.

The challenges and issues seen until now dealt with the forecasting models only. But along with these models there are a few more issues that need to be considered. As the incubation period of COVID-19 is 2–14 days, it is very difficult to identify the patient before the incubation period. Within this period the virus can infect a whole lot of people who come in contact with that person. That leads to our next problem, i.e. tracking of people. It is very difficult to track people who come in contact with the person. Many countries are imposing complete lockdown and shutdown of businesses. But it is very difficult to accurately predict the precise duration of the lockdown. If lockdown is revoked too quickly, then the virus can spread at a faster rate than anticipated.

4.4 RECOMMENDATIONS

The following are recommendations given by WHO to be followed by people all over the world. These people can be categorized as follows:

(i) Citizens
(ii) Suspected and infected patients

4.4.1 Recommendations for Citizens

(i) To maintain hygiene, wash your hands as frequently as possible. Wash your hands with soap and water or use an alcohol-infused hand-wash.

(ii) To stay healthy, maintain social distancing. That means maintaining a distance of at least 1 meter between yourself and the infected person (who is coughing and sneezing)..

(iii) Try not to touch your mouth, nose, and eyes.

(iv) Whenever coughing or sneezing, use tissues or cover your mouth with your bent elbow. Throw away the used tissue in a dustbin immediately after use.

(v) If you are experiencing COVID-19 symptoms such as, fever, cough, or breathing problems, consult your nearest doctor.

(vi) Follow the advice given by the doctor.

(vii) Even if you are experiencing mild symptoms, stay at home and maintain social distancing [9].

4.4.2 Recommendations for COVID-19 Suspected and Infected Patients

COVID-19 is a novel respiratory disease which was first observed in Wuhan, China. It has been observed that most of the patients only experience mild to uncomplicated illness. Fourteen percent of patients actually develop severe symptoms which need immediate hospitalization and oxygen support. Only 5% of the patients need the facilities of the intensive care unit. Severe pneumonia is the most common known diagnosis in COVID-19 patients. Guidelines for suspected and infected patients are categorized into the following sections:

(i) Recommendations for hospital management: adults

(ii) Recommendations and caring for pregnant ladies

(iii) Recommendations for quarantine

4.4.3 Recommendations for Hospital Management: Adults

Early recognition of disease in patients can be helpful. Immediate Infection Prevention and Control (IPC) measures can be taken in order to prevent the condition from getting worse. If patients experiencing severe pneumonia symptoms can be detected at early stages, then proper hospitalization, treatment, and support and care at ICU facilities can be provided to the patient.

Elderly patients with an earlier prognosis of health conditions (cardiovascular complications, diabetes, asthma, etc.) are at a higher risk of catching the infection. These patients can rapidly deteriorate because of their earlier prognosis. Such patients experiencing even the mildest of symptoms should be hospitalized as soon as possible. Close monitoring of such patients is very essential.

Patients who are experiencing mild symptoms but do not require immediate hospitalization can be housed in isolation facilities to prevent the mitigation of the virus. These patients should understand the conditions of the isolation set by the local government and should strictly follow these regulations. If such patients begin to experience worse symptoms, they should immediately contact the hospitals designated for COVID-19 treatment. Counseling such patients is also very important so that they are informed about their condition and any forthcoming situation.

4.4.3.1 IPC Measures

(i) There should be at least one IPC point at the entrance of the hospital. Careful screening of each patient should be done. The suspected patient should be removed from the waiting line and a separate area should be prepared for holding such patients. Primarily these patients should be provided with masks. In the holding area there should be a distance of at least 1 meter between the patients.

(ii) Standardized precautions in all healthcare facilities should be implemented. Standard precautions include the following points:

- Supplies should be provided for hand hygiene (hand-wash, alcohol-based sanitizers, etc.).
- Each healthcare professional should be provided with personal protective equipment (PPE) kits before coming in contact with the patient.
- Bio-waste generated in this time is of huge amounts. There should be a way to dispose the waste materials without causing any side effects.
- Equipment used for testing should be cleaned with a disinfectant.

4.4.4 Recommendations and Caring for Pregnant Ladies

As of now, there is no evidence suggesting that pregnant ladies are at a higher risk of infection. There is a chance of infection if a pregnant lady comes in contact with a person who is already infected. There is high chance of asymptomatic transmission of the disease to pregnant women.

Pregnant women who are suspected of infection or have confirmed infection should be provided with skilled care. Along with the medical care, mental care and psychological aid should also be provided, as the infection could give rise to serious complications during pregnancy.

All IPC measures mentioned earlier should be applied in this case. Consultation with obstetric, perinatal, neonatal, and intensive care experts is very essential. Women who have recovered from COVID-19 should be informed about infant feeding options, and along with that, the IPC measures to be followed. If the mother is severely infected with COVID-19, she should maintain distance from her child. The care of the child can be taken by the guardian or primary caregiver.

4.4.5 Recommendations for Quarantine

Quarantine is recommended when a person is not necessarily sick but who may have been exposed to the virus. There is a difference between quarantine and isolation. Quarantine is the separation of a person before symptoms start to show up. Isolation is separation of an infected person from his/her environment in order to stop the virus spread.

If quarantine measures are applied properly, then it can help in stopping local transmission. If these measures are not applied properly, it can create more sources of contamination.

The period of quarantine is 14 days since the last day of exposure. After that, tests should be performed again. If the test results are positive, then the patient is quickly put into isolation. The abovementioned IPC measures are also recommended in this case [10].

4.5 CONCLUSIONS

COVID-19 is spreading across the globe at an unprecedented rate. This book can help in understanding the basics related to COVID-19 and the forecasting techniques related to it. This book is divided into four main chapters.

The first chapter provides an overview of novel COVID-19. Before getting into the disease and its symptoms, the natural course of a disease is discussed. After that the difference between an epidemic and pandemic is discussed, along with some of the major pandemics witnessed by the world. The next part is the introduction to the novel COVID-19 disease. The last part of the chapter deals with the medical overview, nature, and spread of the disease.

The second chapter deals with data processing and knowledge extraction. Before starting with any kind of analysis, data preprocessing is a very important task. So before diving into data processing, the main task is collection of data from various resources. As social media is nowadays becoming an integral part of lifestyle, huge amounts of data are being generated on this platform. This is one of the many sources of data that is discussed in this chapter. In the actual data processing phase data cleaning is carried out. The last part of the chapter deals with knowledge extraction, as data exists in text files, image files, audio files, and video files as well. Hence the extraction methods applied to each of the data source will be unique.

The third chapter deals with the analytics part of the book, i.e. big data analytics for COVID-19. The first part of the chapter gives an overview of the basic terminologies used in data analytics. For a good prediction, the selection of the parameters plays a very important role. Along with the selection of parameters, the data modeling phase is also very important. Data modeling and the phases included in the modeling are also discussed in detail. The third part of the chapter deals with the techniques available for the analysis of the big data. Various techniques along with a handful of tools are discussed in the last part of this chapter. These tools and techniques can be used to get accurate predictions.

The fourth and the final chapter provides a brief overview of the global scenario through case studies of China, Italy, and the United States. The case studies give the statistics of the current situation in the abovementioned countries. The second part deals with mitigation strategies that can be implemented. The third part deals with issues and challenges faced by the forecasting models. The next part of the chapter deals with recommendations for citizens, patients, and healthcare professionals. This last part concludes with the future outlook.

4.6 FUTURE OUTLOOK

Within the scope of this book, data analytics techniques are discussed and driven by one of the prominent fields known as machine learning. However, the size of the data is increasing with each passing moment. The increasing size of the data will make the existing machine learning techniques and algorithms inadequate somewhere in the near future. It means that there will be a stage where these machine learning algorithms will start underperforming. Hence, in this case, deep learning techniques can be applied. These techniques will be able to handle large amounts of data as the COVID-19 pandemic is witnessed by most of the nations across the world. Still in the initial phase, not much data is available. The shortages of the data lead to inadequate performance and predictions. Hence, more research is required in the ensemble model. In the ensemble model multiple models are trained together in order to improve the efficiency and accuracy of the result.

Nowadays there are a number of sources from which data can be generated. This data is essentially in heterogeneous form. Hence, fusion of this data is required to extract information. In this case cognitive computing is an interesting area which can be explored by researchers. In the future, the size of the data will be huge so cloud-driven analytics can be the next possible area that can be explored. As of now, all the analysis is being done on datasets. But in this we are missing actual real-time data. Also, velocity is missing, which is the rate at which the data is being created and the analysis is being done on that data. Hence, we need models that will be able to accommodate real-time data. Quantum computing is also one of the emerging fields in computer science where storing of information can take a whole new approach. This can be potentially helpful in the analysis as well as in the predictions. On April 22, 2020, WHO made a statement that this virus is going to stay with us for a very long time. As mentioned earlier, this will totally alter the definition of the word "normal" in the coming days. This prediction also needs further investigation to avoid panic among the world's population.

REFERENCES

1. The Novel Coronavirus Pneumonia Emergency Response Epidemiology Team. 2020. The Epidemiological Characteristics of an Outbreak of 2019 Novel Coronavirus Diseases (COVID-19) — China, 2020. *China CDC Weekly* 2(8): 113–122.

2. COVID-19 Surveillance Group. 2020. *Characteristics of COVID-19 Patients Dying in Italy: Report Based on Available Data on March 20th, 2020.* Rome, Italy: Instituto Superiore Di Sanita.
3. Remuzzi, A., Remuzzi, G. 2020. COVID-19 and Italy: What Next? *The Lancet* 395: 1225–1228.
4. Epidemiological Trends of COVID-19 Epidemic in Italy During March 2020. From 1,000 to 100,000 Cases. *Journal of Medical Virol* 2020, April 21. doi: 10.1002/jmv.25908. [Epub ahead of print].
5. COVID, C., COVID, C., COVID, C., Chow, N., Fleming-Dutra, K., Gierke, R., CDC COVID-19 Response Team, Roguski, K. 2020. Preliminary Estimates of the Prevalence of Selected Underlying Health Conditions Among Patients with Coronavirus Disease 2019—United States, February 12–March 28, 2020. *Morbidity and Mortality Weekly Report* 69(13): 382.
6. Centres for Disease Control and Prevention. https://www.cdc.gov/coronavirus/2019-ncov/index.html [Accessed: 25-April-2020].
7. World Health Organization. Coronavirus disease (COVID-2019) situation reports. https://www.who.int/emergencies/diseases/novel-coronavirus-2019/situation-reports [Accessed: 25-April-2020].
8. Centers for Disease Control and Prevention. 2020. Implementation of Mitigation Strategies for Communities with Local covid-19 Transmission.
9. World Health Organization. Coronavirus disease (COVID-19) advice for the public. https://www.who.int/emergencies/diseases/novel-coronavirus-2019/advice-for-public [Accessed: 25-April-2020].
10. https://www.who.int/publications-detail/clinical-management-of-severe-acute-respiratory-infection-when-novel-coronavirus-(ncov)-infection-is-suspected.

INDEX